T'ai Chi
Sensing-Hands

Chen Kung's T'ai Chi Series

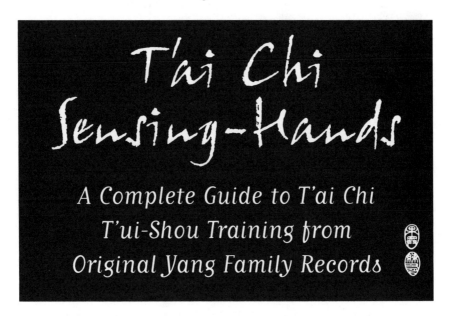

T'ai Chi Sensing-Hands

A Complete Guide to T'ai Chi T'ui-Shou Training from Original Yang Family Records

Translation and Commentary by Stuart Alve Olson

With a Foreword by Jonathan Russell,
Senior Student of Master T.T. Liang

Translatations from
T'ai Chi Ch'uan Tao Chien Kan San Shou Ho Lun (T'ai Chi Ch'uan, Sword, Sabre, Staff, and Dispersing-Hands Combined), by Chen Kung

Disclaimer

Please note that the author and publisher of this book are NOT RESPONSIBLE in any manner whatsoever for any injury that may result from practicing the techniques and/or following the instructions given within. Since the physical activities described herein may be too strenuous in nature for some readers to engage in safely, it is essential that a physician be consulted prior to training.

First Published in 1999 by Multi-Media Books, a division of CFW Enterprises, Inc.

Library of Congress Catalog Number: 98-68620
ISBN: 1-892515-15-1

Distributed by:
Unique Publications
4201 Vanowen Place
Burbank, CA 91505
(800) 332-3330

First Edition
05 04 03 02 01 00 99 98 97 1 3 5 7 9 10 8 6 4 2
Printed in the United States of America.

Edited by Mark V. Wiley
Cover Design by Stuart Olson and Patrick Gross
Photography and Interior Design by Patrick Gross

Dedication

To the memory of Master Jou Tsung Hwa.
His great love for T'ai Chi was unparalleled,
as were his tireless efforts in the creation
of an international center, The T'ai Chi Farm.

His unprejudiced acceptance of everyone, his writings, and above
all his character were truly exemplary.
He will be missed by the entire T'ai Chi world.

I will certainly miss his friendship,
kindness, and support.

Contents

T'ai Chi Sensing-Hands

The Eight Styles of Sensing-Hands

The Four Skills of Sensing-Hands

Acknowledgments

My deepest appreciation to Master T.T. Liang for his many years of helping me through the more difficult parts of Chen's Chinese text, and for all his years of kind instruction and friendship. Not only I, but the T'ai Chi world itself, owes him the deepest gratitude for his numerous contributions to the betterment of T'ai Chi.

Special thanks to my other teacher, colleague, and good friend Jonathan Russell. I thank him not only for writing a foreword to this book, but for his years of support and understanding. He truly deserves the title of Master Liang's Senior Student, as well as his "best" student.

To Master Jou Tsung Hwa, whose untimely death prevented his comments on this book. His encouragement and support of the *Chen Kung's T'ai Chi Series* was always deeply appreciated.

Special thanks to Mr. Pan Li-fan from Shanghai for acquiring the photograph of Master Chen Yen-lin (Chen Kung).

Much appreciation to my friend and student Patrick Gross for his extensive editing and formatting of the entire book, as well as for appearing in the photographs. Although I am truly grateful for the amount of time he devoted to making this work readable and clear, I am more thankful for his persistence in questioning me on the minute details, which have helped render this book a treasure for those who practice Sensing-Hands and martial arts in general.

Many thanks to my friend and student Vern Peterson, who encouraged and helped me begin making the first translation of this book more than eight years ago.

Much appreciation to my friend and student Daniel Dale for appearing in the photographs in the section on the Four Skills of Sensing-Hands.

Many thanks to Mark V. Wiley and Curtis Wong for making this work possible. Without them this would still be one of the many books hidden behind my computer screen.

Others whom I must acknowledge for providing me much encouragement and support are Dr. Poon Yui-koon, Richard Peterson, Lara Puffer, Fred Marych, Larry Hawkins, John Du Cane, and the late Master Oei Khong-hwei.

Lastly, to my son, Lee Jin, whose bright little face makes me constantly seek to do and be better.

The Sung Dynasty Immortal Ancestor, Chang San-feng, Founder of T'ai Chi Ch'uan

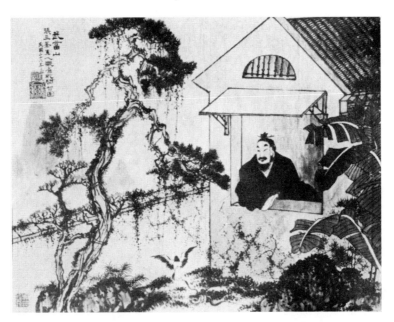

Painting of Chang San-feng watching a bird attacking a snake from his meditation hut on Wu-T'ang Mountain, Hupei Province.

From the simple event of watching a bird attacking a snake, Master Chang formulated the basic premises for the practice of T'ai Chi Ch'uan.

As the snake evaded the strikes of the bird's beak and wings, Master Chang noticed that it would coil and twist away when attacked. When the bird struck the snake's tail, the snake's head would immediately respond. If the bird then attacked the head, the snake's tail would respond. And when the bird resorted to assaulting the snake's body, its head and tail both responded.

After several failed attempts to defeat the snake, the bird surrendered and flew away.

From observing the snake, Chang concluded that employing the entire body as one unit was more powerful than just moving the arms or legs independently, being pliable and relaxed meant greater efficiency and endurance of movement, and that the yielding can overcome the unyielding.

From the insights acquired in watching the bird and snake, Chang was inspired to create the Thirteen Postures of T'ai Chi Ch'uan.

He is also credited with writing the *T'ai Chi Ch'uan Lun (Treatise on T'ai Chi Ch'uan)*, and *T'ai Chi Lien Tan Pi Chueh (T'ai Chi Secret Arts of Refining the Elixir of Immortality)*.

Yang Family Lineage

Yang Lu-chan
Founder of Yang Style T'ai Chi Ch'uan
(1799–1873)

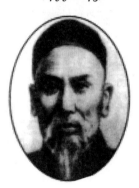

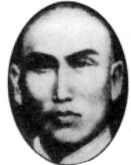

Yang Pan-hou
Eldest Son
(1837–1892)

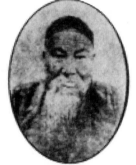

Yang Chien-hou
Second Son
(1839–1917)

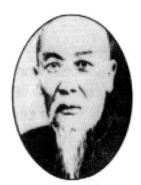

Yang Shao-hou
Eldest Son of Chien-hou
(1862–1930)

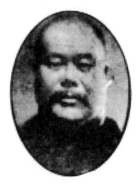

Yang Cheng-fu
Third Son of Chien-hou
(1883–1936)

About the Author
Master Chen Kung

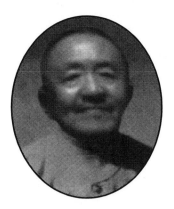

Born in 1906, Master Chen Kung, also known as Yearning K. Chen and Chen Yen-lin, lives and teaches in Shanghai, China. He is a doctor of Chinese medicine and began his T'ai Chi practice at the age of four. His book, *T'ai Chi Ch'uan Sword, Sabre, Staff, and Dispersing-Hands Combined (T'ai Chi Ch'uan Tao Chien Kan San Shou Ho Lun)*, published in 1943, revolutionized many aspects of T'ai Chi practice and theory, especially those concerning his discourses on Intrinsic Energy *(Chin)*, Sensing-Hands *(T'ui-Shou)*, Greater Rolling-Back *(Ta-Lu)*, and Dispersing-Hands *(San-Shou)*.

Chen, however, has remained an enigma to the T'ai Chi world, as he provides no information about himself in his book. The little knowledge known about him came from the late Master Jou Tsung Hwa, who located Master Chen in Shanghai in 1980 and was very impressed with Chen's profound skills with various Intrinsic Energies and with his abilities in Sensing-Hands.

Foreword

In 1943, Chen Kung, a student of the famous T'ai Chi teacher Yang Cheng-fu, published his now classic book *T'ai Chi Ch'uan Tao Chien Kan San Shou Ho Lun.* This book was based on manuscripts Chen had received from the Yang family and his own years of study with the great Cheng-fu. Never before or since has there been such an extensive and complete exposition of the practices and techniques of T'ai Chi Ch'uan. Stuart Olson, in his book *T'ai Chi Sensing-Hands,* is the first to undertake the formidable task of translating into English the section in Chen's original book on *T'ui Shou,* the art of T'ai Chi Sensing-Hands (or Pushing-Hands, as *T'ui Shou* has traditionally been translated into English).

Many concepts and techniques that Chen presents are subtle and esoteric, and translating them into English requires someone who is Western, fluent in translating Mandarin, and deeply familiar with T'ai Chi Ch'uan and all its subtleties. Stuart Olson is uniquely qualified for this task. He is a long-time practitioner of T'ai Chi and had the opportunity to live with Master T.T. Liang in his home in Minnesota for six years.

I met Stuart on my first visit to Liang after he had moved from Boston to St. Cloud, Minnesota, in 1982. "The Monk," as Liang called Stuart because of his interest in Buddhism, was studying Chinese and practicing and teaching T'ai Chi daily with Master Liang—who gave Stuart an original, unabridged edition of Chen's book to translate. I remember well how Stuart would attempt to catch Liang before he escaped to his room for the night and ask him for help in deciphering a section, a word, or a phrase. Stuart was well aware of the privilege of having this text to translate and grateful for Master Liang's inestimable help in doing so. Contained within it are some of the most valuable lessons for anyone interested in T'ai Chi Ch'uan.

Of the many thousands of students that Master Liang, Stuart, and I have taught over the years, very few have grasped the fundamental concept of "quiet minding while investing in loss"—and yet all the techniques in this book are based upon it. Liang would endlessly say, "The more you lose, the more you gain" ("big loss, big gain: small loss, small gain). Though catchy, easy to remember and some may even think naive, this phrase contains the "secret" of T'ai Chi—the key to understanding it.

I recommend that the beginning practitioners of T'ai Chi Sensing-Hands start to understand this concept by thinking of the movements with their partner as a tactile conversation. But the language being spoken is one of movement, sensation, and inner interpretation—not words that are expressed in the basic structure of "Warding-Off, Rolling-Back, Pressing, Pushing, and Neutralizing." In this tactile conversation you want to hear what your partner is physically and mentally expressing, to catch his every nuance. If your head is full of your own ideas, random thoughts, or the desire to "score points," you will never be able to hear what that person is actually expressing or to know what his intention is.

Reaching this state of quiet minding sounds easy, but in practice it is not. If a 300-lb. muscle man is bearing down on you with every intention to knock you over, it's difficult not to erroneously react, not to tense up, not to let your center of gravity float up through the ceiling. But instead you should abide by the *Tan-T'ien* (your center) and quietly listen—so that you will be able to employ the many wonderful lessons this book has to offer.

No T'ai Chi student should be without this book, as the concepts presented, both for the beginner and advanced student, are so valuable and necessary that it should be read over and over again. The contents of this book will make even the most advanced student feel like a beginner. The gratitude given by the Chinese reader of Chen Kung's Chinese version should as well be given to Stuart for this English presentation.

—Jonathan Russell
Senior Student of Master T.T. Liang

Preface

The concepts presented in this work can at times be viewed as vague or complex, and at other times clear or simple in style. This is understandable, and unavoidable, as the subject matter of T'ai Chi Ch'uan is both philosophically and empirically, elementary and complex. The movements and principles inherent within the practice of T'ai Chi may be simple and easy to understand, but they are just the foundation on which is built the "supreme ultimate" art for self-defense, health, wisdom, and longevity.

Large portions of the material presented here have never been accessible to the greater T'ai Chi community—or available at all in the West. The reason, in my opinion, is that it takes years of serious study and practice of T'ai Chi to even approach an understanding of the basic concepts and theories—and not many adherents acquire the longevity or patience to attain this knowledge. The majority of practitioners only learn the basics of the Solo Form of T'ai Chi, and possibly a little of the Sensing-Hands teachings.

Rare are those who are competent in the application practices of Sensing-Hands (*T'ui-Shou*)—commonly referred to as "Pushing Hands"—Greater Rolling-Back *(Ta Lu)*, and Dispersing-Hands (*San-Shou)*. These three exercises are the traditional methods of the Yang Style school for training and developing martial applications and Intrinsic Energies. Even more rare are those who have studied the specific language of the classical T'ai Chi texts presented in the Chinese. Though regrettable, it is not surprising that the more advanced teachings and concepts of this art have not been clearly presented in English.

The majority of material written on T'ai Chi have been either shallow in content or self-serving, in both English and Chinese. T'ai Chi needs to go back to its roots for it to survive the murky existence it has so far endured in the West.

First embraced by the so-called "counter culture" during the '60s, then treated as a curiosity of the martial arts community in the '80s, and presently being cast as a trendy Asian form of health practice—T'ai Chi is so much greater than these limited channels of perception. Without question, T'ai Chi is the physical expression and philosophical culmination of Chinese culture, thought, and philosophy, all set into motion.

I do recognize, however, that T'ai Chi has made a great deal of progress in the West. A handful of accomplished Chinese and Western masters are actively teaching and promoting here, and a number of well-written books, which elucidate the more profound and traditional aspects of T'ai Chi, have been published.

The medical community is also embracing and validating the practice of T'ai Chi as an excellent means for lowering blood pressure, preventing falls, eliminating stress, increasing blood circulation, and providing a better sense of well-being. Many health clinics and hospitals now have T'ai Chi within their curriculum. More and more T'ai Chi centers and schools keep appearing. The media has also been paying a great deal of attention to T'ai Chi within movies, the news, and documentary presentations. All this attention has helped not only in establishing T'ai Chi as legitimate, but firmly lodging it into the consciousness of our population as well.

T'ai Chi suffers the unique problem of being very difficult to organize as a progressive system of learning—as it is devoid of distinct titles, degrees for belts, and certification. All of which, however, I find refreshing and comforting, considering how much we in the West want to commercialize and categorize everything. T'ai Chi, in this regard, has so far proven itself both evasive and non-conforming.

The side-effect to this benefit, however, is the unfortunate proliferation of undeserving teachers attaching "master" to their name. The traditional way to acquire the title of master was bound by the rule that a teacher's students had to bestow this title on him, not teachers giving it to themselves. In China, students would only bestow the title of master on teachers who could demonstrate certain skills—proving their attainment of such a title.

Regardless of the uncomforting and erroneous usage of the title "master," it is a small price to pay for engaging in a system of learning that is predominantly judged personally, and void of the ranking and competitive aspects of so many other related arts. The test, if we should so call it, of T'ai Chi is contained within the practice and skills of Sensing-Hands. No other system of related martial arts bases itself on the premise that the more one learns to lose, the greater the skills for winning—proving to be a difficult concept and goal to accept for the aggressive and strength-minded personality.

Despite recent gains in the exposure of T'ai Chi, its future in our culture should not necessarily be popularized or validated by the media or the medical community. It would be far greater if T'ai Chi, as with any art form, witnesses the development of a western *master-prodigy* of its own—someone who not only exemplifies the highest aspects of the traditional teachings, but creates new boundaries and aspirations as well. Without such a figure, T'ai Chi, I fear, will be doomed to be just another fading trend alongside so many other fading trends in our culture. We desperately need our Mozart, our Einstein, our Picasso, our Yang Lu-chan of T'ai Chi for its sustained growth and long-term acceptance.

Such a person has always been a crucial necessity of every art form in every culture throughout history. To that end, it is my hope that these works from Chen Kung, as well as from the works of other translator-writers, will in some small way play a part, a stepping stone, in aiding the achievement and realization of such a master.

About the Translation

The text is organized just as Chen Kung placed it in the Chinese version. I tried as much as possible to stay true to the Chinese original, but English and Chinese are at times uncooperative with each other. For the sake of readability, I was sometimes compelled to embellish a single character into an entire sentence. The majority of the translation, however, is literal, and to a lesser degree a free translation. Although the translation stays very true to the original, there are a few items I had to either alter or change in order to make the book read easier.

Firstly, the topmost names of the Eight Styles are my creation, as is the name *Eight Styles*. The original names appear in parentheses underneath them. I feel that the names I invented are easier to remember and that they describe the exercises better.

Secondly, the sentence structure for the exercises in the original was very disorganized. I reorganized them so they would be more understandable. Also, in connection with this, the instructions given in the first exercise were to be assumed by the reader in the next exercises. For example, in later exercises the instruction for each person to stand in a Bow Stance was omitted, rather the text simply states "bring the right foot forward." Therefore, I comment where necessary on the omitted or assumed instructions so that the reader will not have to second guess the text.

The section on Eight Styles contained only a few drawings, and they were very difficult to simulate and correspond with the instructions, being unclear and sometimes incorrect. Chen Kung admits this in the original text. For greater clarity, all the drawings have been replaced with detailed photographs.

All the instructions given in the text are for the Right-Style stances, as are all the photographs. All of T'ai Chi is based on right-side movements, the *Yin* side. The Left-Style, or *Yang* side, is only to be practiced when there is a degree of competency with the right side first. This is true even of the Solo Form, Weapons, and likewise Sensing-Hands. Since the Left-Style stances are directly opposite of Right-Style stances, there was no need to either present them with instructional text or photographs. It will be easy enough for practitioners to figure them out when ready to do so.

Also included are photographs for performing the Three Posturings *(High, Medium,* and *Low)* in the section on the Four Skills of Sensing-Hands, Fixed-Stance. There was no need to include these in the section on the Eight Styles, or in the Active-Steps instructions, as the Fixed-Stance photographs clearly show these body levels, and it will be very easy to assimilate and apply the different posturings to the Eight Styles and Active-Steps later as you progress.

The reader should pay attention to two important sections. The first is the material on *Adhering, Joining, Sticking, and Following.* To those who have some experience with Sensing-Hands, this very helpful information will broaden their perspective and possibly increase their skills. To understand and see how these four abilities relate to the postures of Warding-Off, Rolling-Back, Pressing, and Pushing can provide an entirely knew approach to Sensing-Hands practice.

The other important area is comprised of the discussions on *Adhering* and *Sticking* within the Eight Styles instructions. Paying attention to these will also greatly benefit anyone's Sensing-Hands skills. To understand and see how *Adhering* and *Sticking* relate to *Issuing* and *Seizing,* to *Yang* and *Yin,* to Substantial and Insubstantial, and to Pushing and Neutralizing can provide a whole new outlook and approach to Sensing-Hands.

Because of the importance of studying the *Adhering, Joining, Sticking, and Following* section, as well as the specific information on *Adhering* and *Sticking,* I strongly suggest that you read the entire book before attempting to perform any of the exercises. The material presented in each section of this book rely on information from the other sections, so you must have a grasp of what is being said throughout the book.

The smaller text notes within the translated sections are mine—they are not part of the original. I placed them directly into the text for easier reading, rather than using the normal method of placing them as notes at the end of each section or at the bottom of corresponding pages.

Also, I hope you will forgive my seemingly overusage of capitalized and italicized words. I do this to draw attention to important terms—so that it is clear when talking about a principle phrase from the classics or to refer to an Intrinsic Energy.

Lastly, at various instances in his commentaries, Chen Kung refers to the "old and original writings," which had puzzled me when I first translated this work in the 1980s. Since that time, however, a number of treatises from various lineages of T'ai Chi have been released and published in China. Douglas Wile in his *Lost T'ai-chi Classics from the Ch'ing Dynasty* (Suny Press, 1996) has done an excellent job of presenting and researching these texts.

For my purposes, these texts have shown me that Chen Kung had been in possession of at least a few of them—and this was more than fifty years ago. Many of the sentences and ideas used in this book, as well as in *Cultivating the Ch'i, Intrinsic Energies of T'ai Chi Ch'uan,* and the future following volumes on *Ta-Lu* and *San-Shou*—all translations from Chen Kung—contain information and obviously derive from these old, lost treatises (which have recently been revealed to us). This has caused me to believe that I should at some point in the near future cross reference the entire series of Chen Kung, who has drawn his information from very traditional and historical sources—proving again how valuable the information in his book is to the T'ai Chi world.

Sensing-Hands training has a deep relationship to the Intrinsic Energies *(Chin)* of T'ai Chi, and it is highly suggested that the reader refer to my other translated works of Chen Kung—*The Intrinsic Energies of T'ai Chi Ch'uan* and *Cultivating the Ch'i.* These books provide the background knowledge, benefits, purposes, and goals of *T'ai Chi Sensing-Hands.* Without the information in these works many of the terms and concepts presented here might not be readily clear and understandable to the reader.

I also strongly suggest that the reader examine two other books: *T'ai Chi Ch'uan for Health and Self-Defense* by Master T.T. Liang, and *The Tao of T'ai Chi Ch'uan* by Master Jou Tsung Hwa. Both of these works contain a great deal of very important T'ai Chi information. Other suggested reading is provided at the end of this book.

—*Stuart Alve Olson*

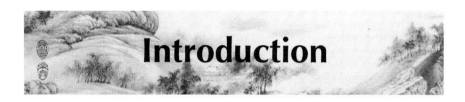

Introduction

Although *T'ui-Shou* has been popularly translated as "Pushing-Hands," I have always felt that this term was misleading to the purpose and essence of *T'ui-Shou*. The Chinese character for *T'ui* is composed of two ideograms. The main radical on the left *(Shou)* simply means a "hand," and the ideogram to its right *(Chui)* means bird.

The character *T'ui* then presents the image of a "bird within the hand," and has commonly been translated with the meanings of "yielding," "pushing something upwards to release it," "to hand over," and "to examine something carefully."

Shou, the other character in the compound of *T'ui-Shou,* also means "hand," but can also carry the meanings of "skill," "effort," and "action." Therefore, *T'ui-Shou* could likewise, and more precisely, be translated as "Sensing-Skills." I feel, however, that the clearest and most appropriate translation for *T'ui-Shou* is that of *Sensing-Hands.*

My reason in foregoing the standard translated term of Pushing-Hands is twofold. Within the Yang Family records we find a story about Yang Chien-hou, the second son of Yang Lu-chan (the founder of the Yang Style system of T'ai Chi). In this story, Chien-hou provides a demonstration of his profound Intrinsic Energy skill of *Interpreting* by showing how he could prevent a sparrow standing on the palm of his hand from taking flight. As the bird attempted to gather momentum by pushing downwards, Chien-hou would hollow his palm, without grasping the bird by any means with his fingers, and thus halted the bird's ability to fly away.

Whether Chien-hou could really perform this feat or not doesn't matter. What this story provides is a wonderful example of *Interpreting Energy,* which is developed through *T'ui-Shou.* And as previously mentioned, the character for *T'ui,* interestingly enough, shows a "bird within the hand." The *Interpreting* ability to accomplish such a feat implies a very heightened sensitivity within Chien-hou's hand. The bird may have attempted to "push," but Chien-hou was able to "sense" the movements and respond to them.

The second reason for translating *T'ui-Shou* as Sensing-Hands is that to use the expression of "pushing" carries the erroneous concept of force and exertion, something which is contrary to T'ai Chi philosophy and practice. The language of any art form is crucial as it can influence our actions greatly. The divergence in perception and meanings of the words "pushing" and "sensing" is very wide. "Pushing" implies a hard and aggressive action, whereas "sensing" implies an action that is cautious and defensive, a type of introspective awareness.

The word "push" does not actually exist anywhere in T'ai Chi terminology, even within the posture translated as *Pushing.* Actually, the name derives from the Chinese term *An,* which means "peaceful, quiet, natural, and effortless." Again, by adding the radical *Shou* for *hand* alongside it the idea of effortlessly restraining something came about. The posture was most likely not translated as Pushing because of the language, but because in application it appears as if that is what is occurring. Pushing in T'ai Chi is more related to the idea of the energy coming off the end of a whip to repel an object than to that of pushing an object away.

Various T'ai Chi Ch'uan classical texts have used the term *Ta-Shou,* and some people have translated this as Pushing, but it should more correctly be translated as "Sparring-Hands," or "Defending-Hands." The term *Ta-Shou* has also had a long association with gesturing or signing with the hands and fingers, or as it is sometimes called "Expressing-Hands."

The hands in T'ai Chi, like the antenna of an insect or the whiskers of a cat, act more as sensors than as instruments of strength. Energy is expressed and issued through them. They are not the source of the energy itself, no more than the tip of a whip is the source of the energy it emits.

Hands in T'ai Chi are simultaneously the receptors of information and the transmitters of responding to that information. As Yang Cheng-fu well related, "Hands? We have hands all over our body, but it has nothing to do with hands." Meaning, our entire body should be perceived as if it were a hand *Interpreting* the actions of an opponent. Likewise, with such a perception, the response could be expressed from any part of the body as well.

With all the above in mind, I choose to use the term *Sensing-Hands*, and from now on that term will be used exclusively.

How to Practice Sensing-Hands

The biggest obstacle any person encounters in taking on the practice of Sensing-Hands is the attitude of wanting to win, to better the person with whom they are practicing. The very premise of all T'ai Chi practical applications for self-defense, however, is in learning "how to lose." Without this intent no one can learn to yield or abide by the *Tan-Tien*. It is absolutely crucial not to let your Sensing-Hands training become a free-for-all wrestling match. Otherwise, you will just be training the *Li* aspects (External Muscular Force) and not *Chin* (Intrinsic Energy).

Train incessantly to learn how to take advantage of your opponent's defects with *using the energy of your waist and legs,* not with your hands and arms. Learn how to lightly touch your opponent, rather than forcefully grabbing him. Learn how to breathe with the movements so that eventually you can *Entice* an opponent with just your breath. These are the most important physical aspects of Sensing-Hands. Pay attention to them and learn to apply them.

Another piece of advice, but not totally necessary, is for beginners to practice with someone of the opposite sex. The reason for this is that a female is by nature *Yin* and has difficulty expressing *Yang* energy. A male is *Yang* by nature, but has difficulty expressing *Yin* energy. By initially practicing together, the female can gain a greater sense of *Yang* and the male can gain *Yin* energy. It will also prevent the practice from becoming too aggressive. When two males first begin training Sensing-Hands, it is easy for aggressive actions to enter into the movements. With two females it is easy for the exercises to become too passive. Initially practicing with someone of the opposite sex balances out the insufficiencies of both partners.

Sensing-Hands is just that, *sensing.* The primary focus is on learning to *Interpret* not only the opponent but, more importantly, yourself. The very term "self-defense" should not be viewed so much as a means of defending yourself against an opponent, but more so as a means of "defense against yourself." In any contest it is usually our own defects, our own mistakes, and our own inability to read a situation that causes our defeat. Sensing-Hands is the means whereby we can overcome our own defects, mistakes, and lack of perception.

In practicing Sensing-Hands do not concern yourself with actually *Issuing* to your opponent; rather, focus on having just the Mind-Intent of doing so. Making use of a playful imagination, rather than a physical aggressive expression. "First in the mind, then in the body," as the *T'ai Chi Ch'uan Treatise* states. Through gradual practice the Intrinsic Energy of your body will start to appear, but this can only occur if you first train the body to be *Yin* (Insubstantial) so that the *Yang* (Substantial) can appear. T'ai Chi is an art that makes full use of *Yin* energy in order to express and produce *Yang* energy, much like the function of a whip.

In Chinese thought, water (a *Yin* substance) is far stronger than a rock (a *Yang* object). Water overcomes everything, yielding overcomes the resistant, soft overcomes the hard, we can see this everywhere in nature. T'ai Chi is simply a means of imitating this *Yin* force of nature. Consider this well when engaging in Sensing-Hands, otherwise your skills and progression will be greatly deterred.

The Three Interpreting Skills of Sensing-Hands

First and foremost, Sensing-Hands develops the ability to *Interpret*. Meaning that the adherent becomes exceedingly sensitive and alert to the actions and intentions of an opponent. This *Interpreting* skill creates the ability to recognize the intent of an opponent in three manners:

1) *Sensing the Actualization.* As the coarsest skill of *Interpreting*, this is where you determine the physical movement of an incoming attack and then Neutralize it. This is like seeing an arrow just as it is shot and being able to evade it.

2) *Sensing the Inception.* In this more refined application, you are able to sense an opponent's initial intent to draw in force in order to attack you, but you close it off before it is released. This is like seeing

the arrow just as it is being drawn back in the bow and then stepping in and preventing the release of the arrow in the first place.

3) *Sensing the Mind-Intention.* In this, the highest aspect of *Interpreting,* you are able to sense the intent in the opponent's eyes before he can physically express any action. Thus, you can choose to defeat the opponent before the bow is even raised—or, on the other extreme, allow the arrow to nearly reach your body before deflecting it.

An interesting effect of acquiring the latter two skills of *Inception* and *Mind-Intention* is that the actions of an opponent no longer appear fast or quick. Your responses, on the other hand, appear fast and quick to him. This is all due to the heightened awareness of the processes of what an opponent has to undergo in order to initiate an attack. Through the skills of *Interpreting,* you can more easily distinguish the inception of an opponent's actions, and thus have the foresight comfort of being there before the attack arrives. "Heading him off at the pass," or not being there at all so that his force lands on nothing, is upsetting to an attacker, who relies on the premise that his attack will meet with something substantial in order to sustain his center of balance.

The underlying factor for acquiring the *Three Interpreting Skills* of Sensing-Hands is *Sung,* the ability to be in a state of relaxation externally while maintaining a heightened sensitivity and alertness internally. *Sung* is the primary basis for all Intrinsic Skills, and without the development and ability of *Sung* there is no T'ai Chi.

When you practice the Solo Form, for example, you may believe that you are relaxed, but in part this is an illusion. You can't know for sure whether you truly have *Sung* or not until you test yourself with Sensing-Hands practice. Our bodies react differently when being touched. Self-protectionism encroaches, as does tension and anxiety. *Sung* is the elimination of these defects.

The Function, Foundation, and Expression of T'ai Chi
Whether you practice the Solo Form *(T'ai Chi Ch'uan),* Sensing-Hands *(T'ui-Shou),* Greater Rolling-Back *(Ta-Lu),* Dispersing-Hands

(San-Shou), Sword *(Chien),* Sabre *(Tao),* or Staff *(Kan),* they must all be rooted in the following three aspects in order to be properly called T'ai Chi:

1) The *T'ai Chi Axis* (or the waist of the body) works as the pivotal axis and foundation of all T'ai Chi movement, providing the very *function* of *Yin* and *Yang* expression in the body. The following two aspects find their use and purpose through the *function* of the T'ai Chi Axis.

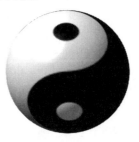

The T'ai Chi Diagram represents the T'ai Chi Waist

2) The *Five Activities* are found in the movements of the feet, the *foundation* of T'ai Chi. The Five Activities are *Advancing, Withdrawing, Looking-Left, Gazing-Right,* and *Fixed-Rooting (Chung Ting),** and they relate to the *Five Elements* (activities) of *Metal, Wood, Fire, Water,* and *Earth.*

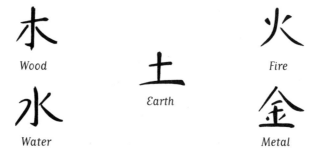

*Normally, the character *Ting* has been translated as Central-Equilibrium. The term *Chung* (middle) *Ting* (balance) can be translated as Central-Equilibrium, or Center of Balance. However, in regards to the Five Activities, just the character *Ting* is used. Keep in mind, it is used as an activity, thus I choose to call it Fixed-Rooting, as that is the function of *Ting*—not a static equilibrium.

3) The *Eight Postures* correspond to the positioning of the hands
and arms, and serve as the *expressions* of T'ai Chi application.
The Eight Postures of *Warding-Off, Rolling-Back, Pressing,
Pushing, Pulling, Splitting, Elbowing,* and *Shouldering* relate
to the *Eight Diagrams* of *Ch'ien (Heaven), K'un (Earth), K'an
(Water), Li (Fire), Sun (Wind), Chen (Thunder), Tui (Valley),* and
Ken (Mountain).

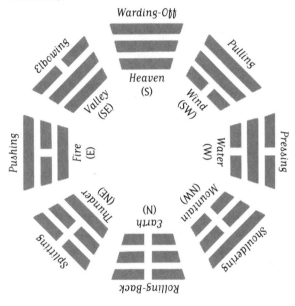

The Eight Diagrams and Corresponding T'ai Chi Postures

The T'ai Chi Axis, the Five Activities (or Elements), and the Eight
Postures represent the *function, foundation,* and *expression* of T'ai
Chi, which also happen to embody the basis for all of Chinese
thought and practices.

Yin-Yang Theory is revealed through the T'ai Chi Axis, *Five
Activities Theory* through the Five Elements, and *Eight Diagram
Theory* through the Eight Postures. By extension, these three aspects
also relate to the concepts of the Chinese philosophy of *San-Tsai—
Heaven, Earth,* and *Man.* The T'ai Chi Axis is representative of
Heaven and the *waist,* the Five Activities of *Earth* and the *feet,* and
the Eight Postures of *Man* and the *hands.*

All of these concepts and philosophies play a very important part in the understanding and applications of Sensing-Hands. Even though one need not go too deep into the study of them to gain the rudimentary skills of Sensing-Hands, there is a definite need to do so to reach the higher level of skills.

The correspondences of T'ai Chi's *function, foundation,* and *expression* to Chinese philosophy were mentioned here to give the reader an overview and introduction to the philosophical tenets of Sensing-Hands, which are all touched upon within the main text of this work.

The Three Divisions of T'ai Chi Practices

As a means of providing another overview of T'ai Chi, the following list of practices shows where Sensing-Hands fits in with the entire system of Yang Style training. This list is for the most part the manner in which Chen Kung's book prescribes the progression of training for T'ai Chi students. Not listed, however, are the additions on theoretical studies on the Intrinsic Energies, T'ai Chi Classics, Essential Principles, and History—which are as equally important as practice itself.

The Three Divisions and Nine Sections of Training

1) Empty-Hand Training consists of learning:
   i) *Ch'i Kung* (Breathing Exercises)
   ii) *Chuang Pu* (Standing Exercises)
   iii) *T'ai Chi Ch'uan* (Solo Form)

2) Two-Person Training consists of learning:
   iv) *T'ui-Shou* (Sensing-Hands)
   v) *Ta-Lu* (Greater Rolling-Back)
   vi) *San-Shou* (Dispersing-Hands)

3) Weapons Training consists of learning:
   vii) *Chien* (Sword Form)
   viii) *Tao* (Sabre Form)
   ix) *Kan* (Staff Drills)

Each of the nine sections can be, and are, complete practices unto themselves. However, the mastery of the Yang Style system of T'ai Chi entails gaining proficiency in all of them.

Other schools of T'ai Chi are not as extensive as the Yang Style. Yang Lu-chan first studied and developed his style from the Chen Style, which is considered the original system of T'ai Chi (although older records suggest that T'ai Chi may have existed far earlier than that of the Chen Style). The other popular systems of Wu Style from Wu Chien-chuan, Hao Style from Hao Wei-jin, and Sun Style from Sun Lu-tang all developed more or less directly from the Yang Style. This is not to say that the other styles are any better or worse than the Yang Style, as each has its special characteristics and focus.*

To a certain degree, each style of T'ai Chi has borrowed and used various exercises and principles described in this work for the basis of their two-person training and practice of Sensing-Hands. Therefore, and please note, *the exercises presented here apply to any style of T'ai Chi.*

Beyond Sensing-Hands

Even though the serious practice of Sensing-Hands will provide you with numerous skills and attainments, it is only one-third of the system for mastery of T'ai Chi practical application. Beyond Sensing-Hands enter the practices of Greater Rolling-Back *(Ta-Lu)* and Dispersing-Hands *(San-Shou)*.

In brief, Greater Rolling-Back concerns itself primarily with the training of Pulling, Splitting, Elbowing, and Shouldering of the Eight Postures—whereas Sensing-Hands focuses primarily on Warding-Off, Rolling-Back, Pressing, and Pushing. Greater Rolling-Back then completes the training of the entire Eight Postures, and is comprised of two main exercises: *Fixed-Stance Greater Rolling-Back* and *Active-Steps Greater Rolling-Back.*

---

*For background history and descriptions of these styles see *The Tao of T'ai Chi Ch'uan* by Jou Tsung Hwa, and *Chinese Boxing—Masters and Methods* by Robert W. Smith.

The third practice, Dispersing-Hands *(San-Shou)*, is an eighty-eight posture two-person form, which in essence ties in the training and applications of Sensing-Hands and Greater Rolling-Back, along with applications from the T'ai Chi Solo Form. It is without question the apex of the art.

Through the long-term practice of these three sections of exercises you will surely come to acquire many of the skills and abilities described as Intrinsic Energies *(Chin)*, which will bring you very near to the mastery of T'ai Chi. Once you have a good familiarity with Sensing-Hands and the T'ai Chi Solo Form, it is recommended that you begin learning both Greater Rolling-Back and Dispersing-Hands. There is no problem in studying and practicing all three sections simultaneously, provided you have the time and means to do so.

Many adherents approach the self-defense aspects of T'ai Chi by first seeking to learn the applications of each posture, which is actually detrimental to the development of T'ai Chi skills. It is far better to concentrate on learning Sensing-Hands, Greater Rolling-Back, and Dispersing-Hands, as these train not only the Intrinsic *(Chin)* abilities for practical use, but even more importantly eliminate the defective and inherent qualities of applying *Li* (External Muscular Force). Through gradual practice, Intrinsic Energy develops and begins expressing itself, which is far stronger and more efficient and exacting than any form of muscular force.

As important as the above practices are, you should also endeavor to study as much as possible. Studying falls into three categories: the T'ai Chi Ch'uan Classics, the Discourses on Intrinsic Energies, and the Twenty-Three Essential Principles of T'ai Chi. The theory of T'ai Chi is just as important as the practice.

Albert Einstein once said, *"Theory without practice is sterile; practice without theory is blind."* This statement is especially true for those seeking to master T'ai Chi. Too many T'ai Chi adherents fall very far from the goal because they have not investigated or examined carefully the above three areas of study. If the ideas and concepts are not in your mind, they can never be expressed in your body. It is absolutely essential to study as well as practice.

Studying with a Teacher

Ko Hung, the famous Taoist of the Six Dynasties period (320 A.D.) wrote in his Taoist classical work the *Pao P'u Tzu* that *"more attention should be given to finding a good teacher, than to finding a method."* Countless people are teaching countless methods. Some are charlatans, and some are genuine. When you find a good teacher, if possible stay with him or her for a long period of time. Don't be like so many present-day adherents who keep jumping from one method and teacher to the next. You will accomplish nothing in doing this other than gaining a smattering of confused information.

On the other hand, there is also nothing wrong in seeking out other good teachers to see what you might add to your body of learning, or to simply compare teaching methods and styles. However, stay with one teacher as your foundation. My teacher, even though he learned from more than fifteen other teachers, stayed with his main teacher for more than twenty years.

In essence, all methods are identical in the end. The art cannot make the artist; rather, it is the artist who makes the art. It is so pointless to think that one method is greater than another, and it is even more absurd to think that the teacher is somehow less important than the method. As the Chinese are fond of saying, "No ivory can come from a dog's mouth." So too, no good student can come from a poor teacher. To be fortunate enough to study with a good teacher greatly outweighs any method you might embark upon.

So if you find a good teacher, study well what he or she teaches you and don't worry about other methods or even other teachers. Move on later if you feel the teacher can take you no further. But do not be like the person who reads two chapters of a book, sets it down, and then moves on to do the same with another book, and another, and another.

That said, it is important to read good books, but don't just read them once and store them on a shelf. Read them several times. I used to read my teacher's book every month, and did so for several years. Each time I gained something new from it. As my practice grew, so did my understanding of what he had written.

T'ai Chi, like all arts and communities of adherents, has its politics, most of which falls into the category of the petty. It is well advised to keep yourself far away from it. Teachers and adherents who go out of their way to speak bad of others more often than not have some personal defect or inner turmoil of their own. No one in this world is perfect, teachers and students alike. Everybody has good and bad points, but always look for the good in others. A Chinese saying runs, *"You can see the faults of others quite clearly, but you cannot see the dirt on the back of your own neck."*

Try your best to stay far away from persons who criticize others. Find a good teacher and good people with whom to practice. Again, another Chinese verse says, *"Be careful of the house you choose, for your neighbors' children will be the greatest influence on your children."* By extension, *"Be careful of the teacher you choose, as his students will be your greatest influence."*

Lastly, practice and study often, yet gradually. This is the only secret. Nothing good is ever accomplished without repetition, whether you practice medicine, write, play golf, paint, or do T'ai Chi. Above all, be patient and allow the practice to gradually become a part of your life, rather than trying to force it on yourself.

T'ai Chi
Sensing-Hands

A Complete Guide to T'ai Chi T'ui-Shou Training
from Original Yang Family Records

Master Chen Kung's Introduction

In the practice of the *Thirteen Posture Boxing (Shih San Ch'uan)*, or the *Square-within-a-Circle Posturing (Pan Chia Tzu)*, the entire body, breath, and mind are all developed and nourished. But in order to advance further, you must learn all of the energies *(Chin)*, such as *T'ing (Listening)*, *Tung (Interpreting)*, *Nien (Sticking)* and *Fa (Issuing)*, and without *Sensing-Hands* these can never be acquired.

Translator's Comments

Thirteen Posture Boxing (Shih San Ch'uan) and the *Square-within-a-Circle Posturing (Pan Chia Tzu)* are older names for T'ai Chi Ch'uan. *Thirteen Posture Boxing* is most likely the original name for this form of martial art, which was first attached within the works of the founder, Chang San-feng, and the *Square-within-a-Circle Posturing* came out of the works attributed to Wang Chung-yueh, a Ming dynasty disciple descendant of Chang San-feng. Other names for T'ai Chi Ch'uan were introduced during its development, such as "Long Boxing," "Cotton Fist Boxing," and "Shadow Boxing," however, T'ai Chi Ch'uan has in present times become the standard term for this art of boxing.

Thirteen Posture Boxing was so named because of the thirteen actions or techniques associated with T'ai Chi movements, which are as follows: 1) Warding-Off, 2) Rolling-Back, 3) Pressing, 4) Pushing, 5) Pulling, 6) Splitting, 7) Elbowing, 8) Shouldering, 9) Advancing, 10) Withdrawing, 11) Looking-Left, 12) Gazing-Right, and 13) Fixed-Rooting.

The first eight postures correspond to the *Eight Diagrams* and the *Eight Directions*. The last five correspond to the *Five Activities* (representing the *Five Elements—Wu Hsing*—of Metal, Wood, Water, Fire, and Earth). Assigning the Five Activities as postures is a misnomer in the sense that the ideas and uses of Advancing, Withdrawing, Looking-Left, Gazing-Right, and Fixed-Rooting are applied within any of the Eight Postures.

For example, in the Rolling-Back posture all five activities are seen in application within the gestures of the posture.
Rolling-Back first begins in a position of Advance with the
forward (right) leg being in a Substantial Stance (a Bow
Stance with weight on the front leg). Next, the body and arms
are brought towards the right side (Gazing-Right). Then the
body is brought back and the weight is shifted into the rear
leg (Withdrawing). Finally, the body is turned to the left
(Looking-Left) and performs the Rolling-Back technique. The
fifth activity, Fixed-Rooting, is applied throughout. There is
no time in the practice of T'ai Chi Ch'uan that this activity is
not applied. In each of the Eight Postures (Warding-Off,
Rolling-Back, Pressing, Pushing, Pulling, Splitting, Elbowing,
and Shouldering) the applications of the Five Activities are
found within their movements.

The *Square-within-a-Circle Posturing* is so named
because within each gesture of any posture the Eight
Directions are strictly maintained. Meaning that, even
though the movements appear to be circular, they are in fact
based on an unseen squareness. For example, when performing the gestures contained within Warding-Off, your
body, waist, and eyes are facing north. The next gesture
moves directly to the northeast, and the final gesture is to the
east. When moving smoothly through these gestures it
appears circular and rounded, but the practitioner, internally,
is moving precisely to a given direction. Briefly stated, the
use of the *square-within-a-circle* technique prevents the
practitioner from creating the defects of "double-floating,"
"double-weighting," and extending one's energy. Again,
these are explained in much greater detail in *The Intrinsic
Energies of T'ai Chi Ch'uan*.

The premise of "the-square-within-a-circle" is entirely
based on the Eight Diagrams *(Pa Kua)* of the *Yi-Ching (Book
of Changes)*, which likewise corresponds to the Eight
Directions (the four cardinal directions of north, south, east,
and west, and the four diagonal directions of northwest,
northeast, southwest, and southeast), and to the Eight Postures

of T'ai Chi (Warding-Off, Rolling-Back, Pressing, Pushing, Pulling, Splitting, Elbowing, and Shouldering).

Body, breath, and mind are a reference to the *Three Treasures (San Pao)*, which is associated with all Taoist theory and practices. In dialectical terms this means that the body is the essence of *Ching*, the regenerative fluids and physical forces of the body; the breath is the essence of *Ch'i*, the vital energy that animates and constitutes the life of a person physically; the mind is the essence of the *Shen*, a person's spirit, which allows one to be mentally and spiritually conscious.*

Chin in translation is "Intrinsic Energy." Since these are also detailed in my book the *Intrinsic Energies of T'ai Chi Ch'uan* I refer the reader to that work, as it would be too lengthy of an explanation here. There are two views on how a person can apply energy in the context of martial art. The first is *Li*, External Muscular Force, which draws its power from tightening the muscles around the bones, storing and drawing that energy from behind the shoulder-blades and back muscles before releasing and striking out, much like the action of hitting with a stick. The second is *Chin*, which stores and draws energy from the bottom of the foot, allowing the entire body to be relaxed. This is similar to the action of a whip or to a snake defending itself from a predator. All of T'ai Chi Ch'uan applications base themselves on this principle. *Chin* is derived from the idea expressed in *Sung*, relaxed, yet sensitive and alert body and consciousness, like that of a cat catching a rat. *Li* is considered in T'ai Chi Ch'uan as not only obstructive to *Chin*, but is quite limited in usage as it is purely a matter of the strong defeating the weak, and the quick defeating the slow. *Chin*, however, is the yielding defeating the unyielding, and the use of an opponent's energy to defeat him. Much like a strong wave or current of water that completely engulfs whatever is in its way.

---

*See my works *Cultivating the Ch'i* and *The Intrinsic Energies of T'ai Chi Ch'uan,* and *The Jade Emperor's Mind Seal Classic* for further information on the *Three Treasures.*

Without the development of the four basic Intrinsic
Energies—*Listening, Interpreting, Sticking,* and *Issuing*—the
application and skills of *Sensing-Hands* will be meaningless
and unproductive. In fact, without having the ability of applying these basic four types of *Chin* there is only the use of
External Muscular Force *(Li).*

Present day T'ai Chi students erroneously begin their *Sensing-Hands*
practice with just the *Fixed-Stance (Ting Pu) Four Skills (Szu Shou)* exercise—consisting of Warding-Off *(Peng),* Rolling-Back *(Lu),* Pressing *(Chi)*
and Pushing *(An)*—as their sole initial training of *Sensing-Hands,* being
unaware of the initial exercises for correct *Sensing-Hands* training.

First you must practice the methods of *Single-Hand, Push and
Neutralize Sensing-Hands,* then the methods of *Two-Hand, Level
Circular Stick and Adhere Sensing-Hands,* and also the methods of
Two-Hand, Push and Neutralize Sensing-Hands and *Two-Hand, Roll-
Back and Neutralize Sensing-Hands,* and so on. You must begin your
training by investigating these *Sensing-Hands* styles. Afterwards you
can learn and practice the *Four Skills in Fixed-Stance* style.

Therefore, the very foundation of any *Kung-Fu* lies in practicing the
fundamental steps and repetitiously enduring them over a long period of
time. For when it becomes necessary to approach an opponent, you must
be capable of seeking out the shortcuts unconsciously. Train with one
hand first and then seek to attain the ability of using both hands. In the
end you will be able to make use of the *Four Skills (Szu Shou)* without
thought. But if you just start with the *Four Skills* you will be unable to
clearly distinguish them. You must understand and know these (eight
fundamental) types of *Sensing-Hands* training procedures.

Translator's Comments
The use of the term *"Kung-Fu"* here is not meant to imply that
these exercises are associated with the hard styles of *Kung-
Fu.* In this instance, *Kung-Fu* is meant as "skillful effort" or
"accomplished skill."

Seeking out the shortcuts unconsciously means that
your skill will be as such that your ability to *Listen (Ting),*

Interpret (Tung), Stick (Nien), and *Issue (Fa)* will occur unconsciously when confronted by an opponent. Through practice
you will be able to sense your opponent's Substantial and
Insubstantial aspects, you will intuitively know the best line
of defense, and how to affect and take advantage of their
defective aspects.

This is no different than a person in their youth who undergoes the
learning procedures of writing books. If in the beginning they do not dis-
cipline themselves in the elementary by copying the individual characters, how could they ever hope to write a book in the future? Thus, the
error is created in the beginning by those who also do not practice the
Single-Hand exercise of *Sensing-Hands.*

If you could put the details of these original procedures and methods into practice, drilling them one by one until adeptness is achieved,
you could then afterwards set to work an earnest effort for the training
of the *Four Skills.* This would then result in your ability to clearly distinguish and analyze the individual gestures of the *Four Skills.*

Moreover, the waist and legs must also apply the intent and energies of *Adhering, Sticking, Joining,* and *Following,* bringing perfect
accord to your actions. By being open and expanded you can acquire
naturalness and will be able to avoid the defects of applying brute force
(Li), rather you will be able to follow both the movements and responses
of the opponent. Then you will have completed the foundation of the
Kung-Fu for *T'ai Chi Ch'uan.*

Translator's Comments
See the section in this work titled *An Explanation of Sticking,
Adhering, Joining, and Following; Opposing, Leaning,
Discarding, and Resisting.*

Below are given the descriptions of the fundamental procedures for
each of the *Fixed-Stance Sensing-Hands* styles.

The Eight Styles
of Sensing-Hands

(The Individual Styles of Fixed-Stance T'ui-Shou)

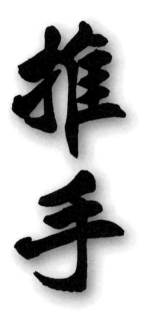

Translator's Preliminary Instructions

In all of T'ai Chi, many specialized terms and phrases are found. Some characters used in the T'ai Chi Classical texts were invented to cloak their actual meanings, others are simply obscure usages, and still others were designed as catch phrases or words that embodied a great deal of meaning. The phrase *"using the energy of the waist and legs"* needs further clarification here so that the instructions in the exercises can be followed more easily. All the other important phrases and terms are defined within the text, but *"using the energy of the waist and legs"* deserves further preliminary explanation as it is fundamental to Sensing-Hands training.

The *function* and *foundation* of all T'ai Chi takes place in the waist and legs, not in the arms and hands. Arms and hands are but the *expression* of T'ai Chi.

The *T'ai Chi Ch'uan Treatise* states:

> The energy is rooted in the feet, issued through the legs, directed by the waist, and appears in the hands and fingers.
>
> The feet, legs, and waist must act as one unit so that whether Advancing or Withdrawing you will be able to obtain a superior position and create a good opportunity.
>
> Failure to obtain a superior position and create a good opportunity results from the body being in a state of disorder and confusion.
>
> To correct this defect, adjust the waist and legs.

These statements clearly express the importance of *"using the energy of the waist and legs."*

The term "energy" in this context is referring to Intrinsic Energy *(Chin)*, not External Muscular Force *(Li)*. Since the foundation of all movement in T'ai Chi originates in the feet, the Five Activities of Advancing, Withdrawing, Looking-Left, Gazing-Right, and Fixed-Rooting come into play through the movements of the waist and legs. *"Using the energy of the waist and legs"* then refers to both Intrinsic Energy and the Five Activities.

The Enticing and Neutralizing Circles

This section provides an example of the *Enticing* and *Neutralizing Circle* movements found in all the Sensing-Hands exercises. These instructions are provided here not only because of their importance to the exercises but also because they clearly show the principle of *using the energy of the waist and legs.*

In this example, the person being Enticed *(B)* is in a Warding-Off position with his left arm held out in a shoulder level half-circular-shape, with the weight of his body centered over his forward (right) leg—(see Photo 1).

A   B

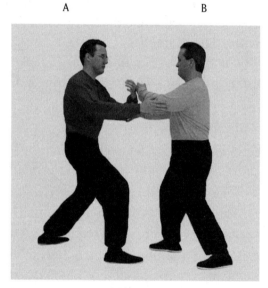

Photo 1

In the instructions for all the Sensing-Hands exercises, directions call for *A* and *B* to face each other standing in Bow Stances with their right legs forward—the Right-Style stance. An important aspect of any Bow Stance is to make sure that the forward foot, specifically the outer edge side of the foot, is placed pointing directly ahead, with the toes then slightly turned inward. The foot has a natural curve, and if the toes were pointed straight ahead this would cause a slight pinching of the buttocks, and make it more difficult to attach your foot to the ground. The rear leg, at shoulder-width distance, should be positioned at a 45-degree angle, and about two foot lengths behind the forward leg. See pages 148–49 for illustrations showing *A* and *B*'s Bow Stances in relationship to the *Three Positionings* and *Three Posturings*.

When being Enticed, the movement leading into Pushing, *B* rises in the forward leg (an Advancing activity) and turns his waist to the right (Gazing-Right—see Photo 2), and then brings it back to the front (Looking-Left—see Photo 3), and sinks. As a result of *B*'s waist and leg movements, his left arm makes a small circling gesture intended to Neutralize the initial Enticing movements of the opponent *(A)*. In this example, *B*'s gesture is properly called the *Neutralizing and Warding-Off Circle;* however, this circling gesture is simply referred to in the exercises as either the Neutralizing Circle or the Warding-Off Circle.

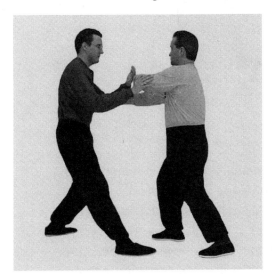 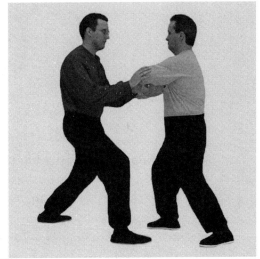

Photo 2   Photo 3

Next, as the opponent *(A)* shifts forward to Push (see Photo 4), *B* rises up slightly in his forward leg, shifts back to the rear leg, and then sinks his weight into it. This rise, shift backward, and sinking movement comprises the activity of Withdrawing, and causes *B*'s arm to rise up and then down to solar plexus level. At no time in these movements, however, does his arm move independently from the rest of his body. It is the movements of his waist and legs that are expressed in his arm, which is circled to the right and then back and down. Likewise, at no time does his body just shift to the rear leg without first *rising,* then *shifting,* and then *sinking.* To do otherwise can cause the defects of *leaning* or *bending* the upper body.

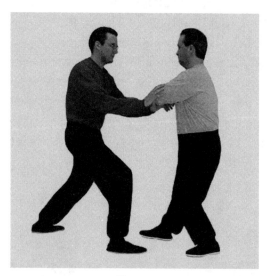

Photo 4

By following the above directions, *B* is *using the energy of the waist and legs,* specifically the movements of the Five Activities, to disrupt the energy of *A's* Pushing. In *rising* and *turning* his waist, *B* uses the activities of *Advancing, Gazing-Right,* and *Looking-Left.* When *rising, shifting* backward, and *sinking* his legs, he uses the activity of *Withdrawing. Fixed-Rooting* is part of every movement.

When describing the movements of the Five Activities in terms of *rising, shifting, sinking, turning,* and, later, *stepping,* the instructions are referring to what is called the *Five Operations.* In fact, all the instructions and commentaries in this book rely on using the ideas of the Five Activities, and their inherent Operations, to describe and teach the movements of the exercises.

In correctly employing the Five Operations of turning your waist, stepping, rising, shifting, or sinking, many situations and opportunities for employing the Intrinsic Energy of *Neutralizing* or some other type of energy can occur. The object of *A*'s Pushing was to uproot *B*, but *B*'s Withdrawing activity causes *A*'s energy to first go up and slightly over to the side, then back and then down, which disrupts the strength in his elbows, thus destroying his intent and line of incoming energy.

Issuing and Neutralizing

In attempting to Push, *A* must also correctly use his waist and legs to utilize the Intrinsic Energy of *Issuing*. The *energy of the waist and legs* applies to *Issuing* as described in the following verse from the *T'ai Chi Ch'uan Treatise:*

> *"The energy is rooted in the feet, Issued through the legs, directed by the waist, and appears in the hands and fingers."*

When you are Pushing, the energy is drawn from the rear foot. It really has nothing to do with any forceful use of the hands, as they just express that energy. This is like a whip in which the handle is your foot, the lash of the whip your waist and leg, and the energy coming off the tip of the whip your hand and fingers. In this analogy, the energy, created in the handle, passes through the lash of the whip, which is relaxed and soft, and appears in the tip. It is because the lash of the whip is relaxed and soft that the energy is able to pass through, and why it is described as *appearing* in the tip. So it should be with your body as well when *Issuing*.

When practicing Pushing in Sensing-Hands, there must first be a Withdrawing activity into the rear leg in order to *Receive* the energy of the opponent, along with a slight Looking-Left to disrupt his line of energy (see *A* in Photo 2). Once this is accomplished there must then be a Gazing-Right activity to realign the waist and legs, immediately followed by an Advancing activity of *rising, shifting* forward, and *sinking* into the front leg (to gain a superior position for Pushing—see *A* in Photo 3).

A's initial Withdrawing and circling movement—called the *Enticing Circle*—coincides with *B*'s *Neutralizing Circle* (described above). The Advancing activity of using the Operations of *rise, shift* forward, and *sink* is similar to driving over a speed bump, and is meant to disrupt the balance and energy of the opponent *(B)*. Withdrawing, then, is like driving over the speed bump in reverse.

Lastly, with arms and hands relaxed, you *rise* upwards off the rear foot to *Issue,* but do not rise completely upwards, otherwise you will create the defects of *double-floating* and *leaning.* Instead, retain the intention when *rising* that there will be a *sinking* or seating of the body once the Push is being executed. This is the T'ai Chi principle of *always keeping something in reserve* (see *A* in Photo 4).

Summary of A and B's Movements

From the preceding instructions, the relationship of movements between the person who is Enticing and Pushing *(A)* and the person Neutralizing and Warding-Off *(B)* can now be summarized.

In terms of the Five Activities and Five Operations, for example, *A* Entices to Push by using the Activities of *Withdrawing, Looking-Left, Gazing-Right,* and *Advancing.* He accomplishes his Enticing and Pushing movements by employing the following Operations: he first *rises* in his forward leg, *shifts* to the rear leg while *turning* left, then *sinks* and *turns* back to the right and front, and then *rises* again, *shifts* the body forward, and *sinks* into the forward leg in order to *rise* off the rear foot, Push *(Issue),* and then *sink* again.

B, meanwhile, uses the Activities of *Advancing, Gazing-Right, Looking-Left,* and *Withdrawing* in order to Neutralize and Ward-Off. He accomplishes his Neutralizing and Warding-Off movements by employing the following Operations: he first *rises* in his forward leg and *turns* to the right, *turns* back to the left and front, and *sinks* into his forward leg (Warding-Off) before *rising* again, *shifting* to the rear leg, and then *sinking* into it to Neutralize the extent of *A*'s Push.

Although these examples of *A*'s and *B*'s movements are summarized in a couple of paragraphs, the instructions are by no means simple and easy to understand in one reading. By using the terms of the Five Activities and Five Operations to describe the movements, however, the directions are able to pack in a tremendous amount of descriptive information in a relatively few amount of words. So when the instructions call for you to *Advance* from the rear to the forward leg, you will then know that this activity implies using the operations of *rising, shifting* forward, and *sinking.*

I have gone into such minute detail here so that the simpler instructional comments within the actual Eight Styles and Four Skills exercises will make more sense, and that you will possess the assumed knowledge of what is being said.

As you will come to see, the Withdrawing and Enticing, Advancing and Neutralizing movements are fundamental to the Sensing-Hands exercises. The Enticing and Neutralizing Circles are the building blocks from which all the gestures and changes in the various exercises occur.

By describing *using the energy of the waist and legs,* the movements of the Sensing-Hands exercises can be seen as generating from the waist and legs—and not from the arms, which primarily follow the movements of the waist and legs.

The following list shows the variations of movements within each of the Five Activities and Five Operations:

The Five Activities

Advancing: to shift, sink, or step forwards.

Withdrawing: to shift, sink, or step backwards.

Looking-Left: to turn or shift leftwards.

Gazing-Right: to turn or shift rightwards.

Fixed-Rooting: after any movement the body must be relaxed and the root in the feet must constantly be reestablished.

The Five Operations

Two types of *Rising:* rear leg and front leg—with the body facing any of the Eight Directions.

Two types of *Sinking:* rear leg and front leg—with the body facing any of the Eight Directions.

Four types of *Shifting:* forward, backward, leftward, or rightward.

Two types of *Turning:* left and right.

Five types of *Stepping:* stepping forward, stepping back, stepping left, stepping right, and repositioning step (Slide Step or Change Step).

Interpreting Energy and the Purpose of Sensing-Hands Training

The central and most important purpose of these exercises is to train *Interpreting Energy*—and not how to express the *Neutralizing* or *Issuing* energies.

In Sensing-Hands *(Ta-Lu* and *San-Shou* as well), the idea is to learn how to *Interpret* the movements and changes of the opponent, and, just as importantly, how to sense your own defects. The *T'ai Chi Ch'uan Classic* says, *"Through knowing yourself, you can know others."* *Interpreting* should be applied first to yourself, and then with an opponent.

Sensing-Hands does not mean *Issuing-Hands.* The exercises are designed to develop *Interpreting Energy,* so to first see clearly the opportunities for expressing the *Six Energies* of *Adhering, Sticking, Enticing, Neutralizing, Seizing,* and *Issuing.* This is accomplished by being able, in a relaxed and slow manner, to clearly distinguish the separate purposes of the Five Activities of Advancing, Withdrawing, Looking-left, Gazing-Right, and Fixed-Rooting, and to refine the Four Skills of Warding-Off, Rolling-Back, Pressing, and Pushing, along with Neutralizing, for properly executing the potential of them, not their kinetic expression.

Every gesture in Sensing-Hands (as well as in *Ta-Lu* and *San-Shou)* is designed to be practiced with the idea that each are being neutralized before they are actually expressed in terms of knocking the opponent over. The exercises in themselves are a stalemate of joined movements. To practice otherwise, with the idea of winning and actually *Issuing,* destroys the very cause for learning how to *Interpret. Issuing* will come later. It will develop without your expressing it in the exercises.

Within *The Intrinsic Energies of T'ai Chi Ch'uan* book, frequent references are made to "using the energy of the waist and legs, *along with the Ch'i and Mind-Intent."* In the Four Skills of Sensing-Hands, and in all the preliminary exercises building up to it, only the *energy of the waist and legs* is used. The kinetic expression of *using the Ch'i and Mind-Intent* is never applied, only its potential use is sensed and developed through the skill of *Interpreting.*

First Style

Single-Hand Sensing-Hands

(Single-Hand, Pushing and Neutralizing T'ui-Shou Method)

Instructions for Right-Style Training
Fixed-Stance
High Posturing, Enclosed Stance

Starting Position

Both players stand opposite of each other (*A* stands to the left, and *B* to the right). Each player brings their right foot forward one step, with both in Right-Style Bow Stances. The left hand and arms of each player are made into half circular shapes, with the backs of the left hands positioned together so that they mutually perform Warding-Off. The right hands are extended outwards with the palms facing forward.

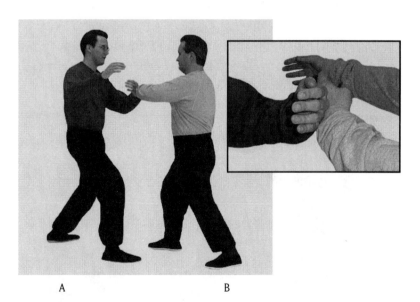

A   B

Translator's Comments

The left elbows should be slightly dropped, but not so much as to be collapsed. The wrists and fingers should be on a smooth line, not with fingers curled or straightened too excessively. Each player should gaze directly at the other. Do not let the eyes look down at anytime during the exercise. *Suspend the head* and *sink the shoulders*. Keep the back straight with the *Wei-Lu* (tail bone) slightly drawn down and under the buttocks.

In this exercise, *A* is *Adhering* and *B* is *Sticking* because *A* will perform Pushing and *B* will be Neutralizing. When the roles reverse, *B* will be *Adhering* when Pushing, and *A* will be *Sticking* when Neutralizing.

The reasons for holding the right hand and arm outwards are threefold: 1) This trains the arm to be in a ready offensive position. 2) It aids in the development of *Sung*—relax in T'ai Chi does not mean collapse. 3) It also aids in *raising the back and hollowing the chest*, so that you don't commit the errors of *leaning* and *bending*. Letting the arm hang will disrupt your *Shen* (Spirit of Vitality), as the entire body must be active and alert

A's Enticing Circle and Pushing

A uses his left hand to perform Pushing, with the intent of Pushing out until such time that he reaches the region near *B*'s chest. When this is to occur, *A* first turns his left palm to the left and then over in a small circling gesture, so the left palm is made to face directly opposite *B*'s heart, *A* then continues Pushing directly forward.

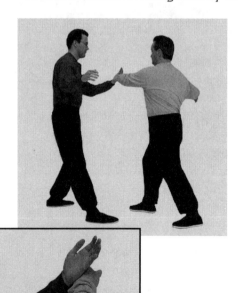

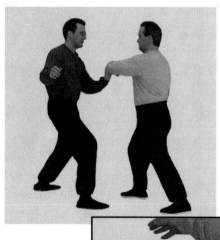

A is Sticking   *A is Adhering*

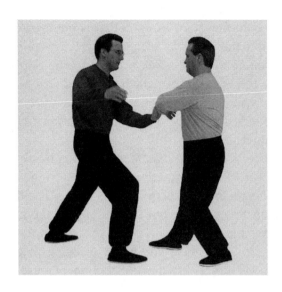

Translator's Comments

Please refer to the preliminary instructions. *A*'s Push should follow the movements as described in that section—starting with the Enticing Circle. The important factor that was not described in that section, however, is the positioning of the hands. In this exercise, *A* starts out with the back of his left hand touching the back of *B*'s left hand. When *A* then performs the Enticing Circle, he turns his hand over when adjusting his waist and legs back to face the opponent (the Gazing-Right movement).

In this and in all the following exercises, when *A* or *B* is about to Push, the back of the Pusher's hand is first attached to the back of the Neutralizer's hand. This means that the person who will be Pushing first *Sticks* to the opponent's hand, then when making the Enticing Circle movements, turns his hand over and *Adheres* to the opponent's hand to Advance and begin the Push (see insert photographs on the preceding page).

When touching the opponent with the back of your hand, you are *Sticking*. When touching the opponent with your fingertips and palm facing the opponent, you are *Adhering*.

When Pushing with two hands, as in the other exercises, the Pusher, *A* for example, starts out *Sticking* with his left hand to the back of the Neutralizer's left hand (except in the *Second* and *Eighth Styles,* in which he *Sticks* his right hand to the opponent's right hand), and *Adheres* with the opposite hand near the opponent's elbow. See instructions under the *Second Style: Pushing & Warding-Off* for further information.

Once you have *Adhered* to the opponent's hand, you complete your Push according to the following three principles: 1) Touch the back of the opponent's wrist and hand with your fingertips only, do not use the butt of the palm as this will reveal too much energy and likewise add tension to the exercise. 2) Have the Mind-Intent of being pulled in, like magnets attracting you into the opponent, not necessarily that you are Pushing. This will likewise eradicate a great deal of tension in your hands and arms, and it will make it harder for the opponent to detect your Pushing. 3) Have the Mind-Intent of directing the Pushing towards the middle of the opponent's chest, otherwise the movements will become sloppy and without precision.

B's Neutralizing Circle and Rolling-Back

B first circles the arm and waist to the right, then shifts directly into the rear leg, seating his waist and relaxing the coccyx region, with the body moving down into a slight squat. *B* Neutralizes, shifting back and down, until *A*'s energy is interrupted.

Translator's Comments

For instructions in Neutralizing, also refer to the preliminary instructions. Remember that *B*'s Neutralizing Circle coincides with *A*'s Enticing Circle.

In a brief summary of the movements, *A* Withdraws into the rear leg, Looks-Left, Gazes-Right, turns the left hand over to *Adhere,* then Advances into the front leg to Push. *A* has then performed the Enticing Circle and Push.

B, meanwhile, Advances, rising in the front leg, Gazes-Right, Looks-Left and sinks, then Withdraws into the rear leg until the energy of the Push is interrupted. *B* has performed the Neutralizing Circle and has Withdrawn into the rear leg—and is now in the position to perform Rolling-Back.

In connection with this, when Neutralizing it is very important to have the Mind-Intent to act as if you are pulling in the opponent's Pushing energy, as if it were magnetic. This perception will not only take away any tension of the Pushing, but will increase your ability not to resist.

B then turns his waist just to the left corner, bringing his left hand along jointly towards the left side, turning it over circularly (a Rolling-Back gesture), using the energy of the waist and legs.

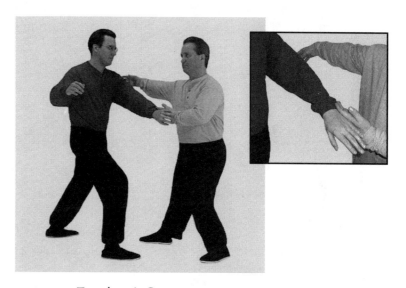

Translator's Comments

When Rolling-Back, it is very important to remember not to turn the waist any further than the immediate corner. Also, when turning (Looking-Left) do not draw the left elbow towards the back, nor raise it. When turning your waist to the left, just turn the hand over—don't do anything else. The elbow will automatically drop slightly, which is precisely what you want to have happen.

When turning over the hand, make sure of two things: 1) Do not press down on the opponent's wrist or hand, just lightly

Stick. 2) Roll over the hand—and do nothing else—such as raising it up and back down again. 3) After turning the hand, make sure the back of your fingers, predominantly the thumb, index, and middle fingers, are on the back of the opponent's palm and fingers, not on his wrist or forearm. This should happen naturally if you just turn over your hand as your waist and legs turn your body to the corner (Looking-Left).

Return to Starting Position
After *B*'s Rolling-Back, *A* initiates a Looking-Left movement into a Warding-Off position. *B* then turns his waist by Gazing-Right and Adhering his left-hand fingers to *A*'s left wrist and hand. Both *A* and *B* then adjust their weight into the front legs, with *B* turning his left palm over to Stick. They are then back in the Starting Position.

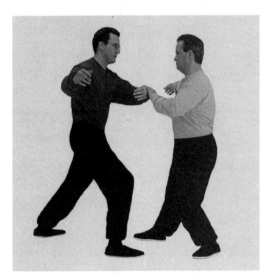 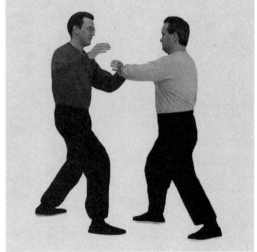

B's Enticing Circle and Pushing,
and A's Neutralizing Circle and Rolling-Back

B now changes to perform the Enticing Circle, Pushing, and Advancing towards the front. A then changes to perform the Neutralizing and Rolling-Back movements, which are identical to the above gestures.

The preceding instructions are for the *Right-Style of Pushing and Neutralizing.* There is also the *Left-Style of Pushing and Neutralizing,* wherein both players mutually bring their left foot forward one step, but this time bring the backs of the right hands together, mutually Warding-Off. This method is identical to the above gestures, except that the turning [Rolling-Back] after the Neutralizing is towards the right corner.

Translator's Comments

Since the Enticing Circle and the Neutralizing Circle apply within all the following Sensing-Hands exercises, *Left-* or *Right-Style* stances, the details will not be repeated unless a new technique or gesture is being called for.

It is well advised to earnestly practice this *Single-Hand Sensing-Hands* exercise so that these principles can become part and parcel of your training and skill.

FIRST STYLE

Single-Hand Sensing-Hands

Enclosed Stance Sequence

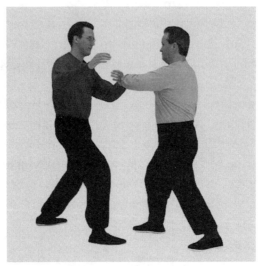

A   B

Starting Position

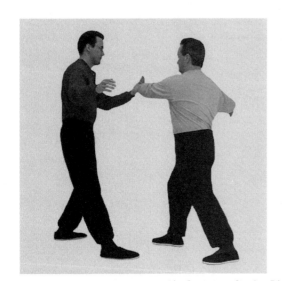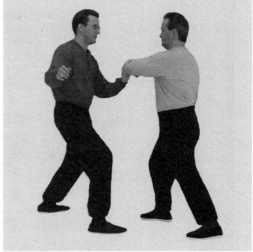

A's Enticing Circle, B's Neutralizing Circle

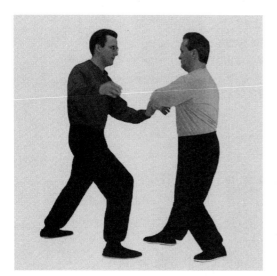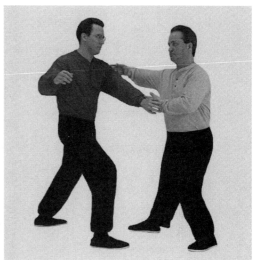

A's Pushing, B's Rolling-Back

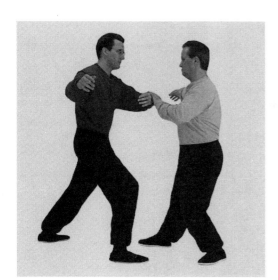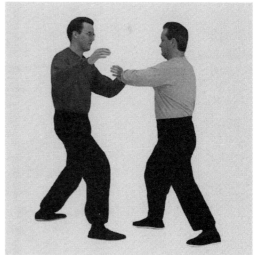

A's Looking-Left to Starting Position,
B's Gazing-Right and Advance to Starting Position

B now performs A's movements.

Pushing & Warding-Off

(Two-Hand, Level-Circular Stick and Adhere T'ui-Shou Method)

Instructions for Right-Style Training
Fixed-Stance
High Posturing, Enclosed Stance

Starting Position

Both players stand opposite of one another, each bringing their right foot forward one step. A places the back of his right hand against the back of B's right hand and wrist to perform the Enticing Circle. The left-hand palm Adheres near B's right elbow.

B brings his right hand and arm out into a Warding-Off position, making the arm into a half-circular shape, and has his left palm Adhere near A's right elbow.

Both players are standing in Right-Style Bow Stances.

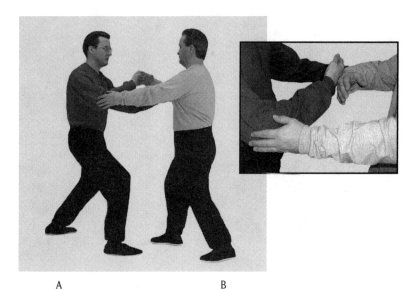

A   B

Translator's Comments

Although A and B start out in *Sticking* positions, A performs the Enticing Circle to move into Pushing and so must turn his hand over to *Adhere*. Since A will be Pushing with the purpose of uprooting B, he must have the intent of *Adhering*. B will be attempting to Neutralize A's intent and must therefore apply *Sticking*. When first learning these exercises, discriminating between *Sticking* and *Adhering* may prove to be difficult, so you need not overly concern yourself with practicing them. As your Sensing-Hands skills improve, however, these types of intents and energies will be of great import.

Also note that the instructions use the term *"near"* for *Adhering* and *Sticking* to the opponent's arm. This is extremely important. To place your hand and palm directly on the elbow and wrist joints of the opponent will create two primary defects. The correct manner is to place the length of the fingers and fingertips on those areas.

The two defects referred to are as follows: 1) If the palm butt is placed directly onto the elbow and wrist joints, the opponent will be able to feel too much of your energy, and will thus be able to *Interpret* it and use it against you. 2) Your own hands and arms will create tension from wrongly placing the butt and palm of your hand on the joints of the opponent. When Pushing, the arm will be stiffened and the wrists and palms will become insensitive. Remember, the *T'ai Chi Ch'uan Treatise* says, *"the energy will appear in the hand and fingers."* It does not state or imply that the energy appears in the *palms* or *palm butts*.

Correctly, you want to apply a light and sensitive touch so to detect the defects and movements of the opponent. This is how to begin developing *Interpreting* energy. Apply any tension in your hands and you will sever your ability to feel and sense, and so obstruct your *Interpreting* ability.

A's Enticing Circle and Pushing

After the Enticing Circle, A performs Pushing with both hands towards B's chest, with the legs ending in a Bow Stance.

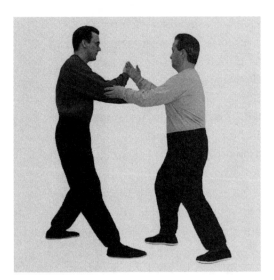 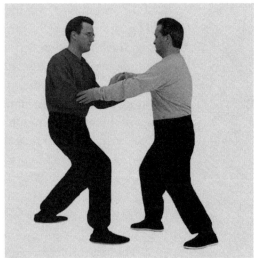

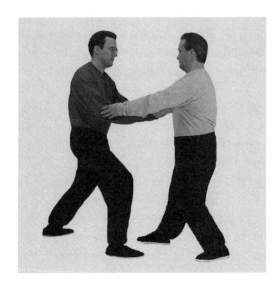

Translator's Comments

When Pushing, begin by making the Enticing Circle as mentioned in the *First Style*. However, since you are now using two hands to Push, you turn over your right hand when circling back to the right (Gazing-Right)—which moves from a *Sticking* position into an *Adhering* one. The left hand is already in the proper *Adhering* position, with the fingers attached near the opponent's elbow. After shifting to your rear (left) leg and circling, shift back into the front leg (Advance) to complete your Push. Remember to draw the energy of the Push from the bottom of the rear foot.

Also, and this is very important, the energy of the Pushing should come through your left hand and be directed into *B*'s right elbow.

B's Neutralizing Circle and Warding-Off

When *A* Entices, *B* Neutralizes *A* by first circling the right arm and waist to the right and then back into Warding-Off. Then when being Pushed, *B* Withdraws to the rear leg and circles the arm towards the left side, downwards, and back—seating the waist, relaxing the coccyx, and seating the legs. The left leg is now Substantial, the right leg Insubstantial, with the center of balance placed directly on the left leg. *B* performs Neutralizing until such time that *A*'s energy is exhausted, but does not turn beyond the immediate corner.

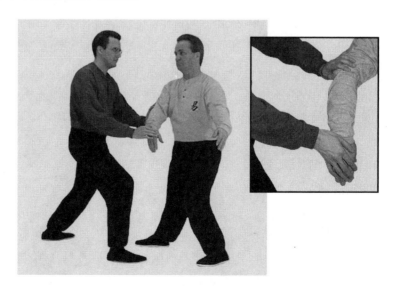

Translator's Comments

When being Pushed, follow the same waist and leg movements as in the *First Style*—except that in this exercise you are Neutralizing with you right arm instead of your left.

After performing the Neutralizing Circle with your right arm, Withdraw into the left leg and continue Neutralizing by making a turning gesture to the left. When going to the left side do so jointly with the shifting back and turning of the waist, but only turn so far as to bring the waist to the immediate corner. When being Pushed, your right arm moves from a Warding-Off position when circling left (Looking-Left) into a Pushing-like position when turning back to the right (Gazing-Right). This circling movement is called for because the opponent has put the energy of his Pushing into your right elbow, and your circling will disrupt and Neutralize it. When you turn your waist and arm back to the right, drop your right elbow so that when you turn back to the right you can end up *Adhering* your hands to the opponent's right hand and elbow. Then Advance into the forward leg so that you can perform the Enticing Circle and Pushing movements. When shifting to the Starting Position, however, turn the right hand over to *Stick* so that you can then perform the Enticing Circle.

Return to Starting Position

A and B turn their waists to face each other again, so they are each centered and upright. Both players have now returned to the starting position, where B can then perform the Enticing Circle and move into Push.

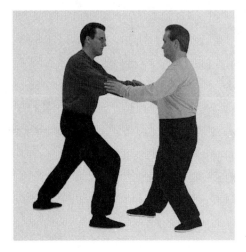 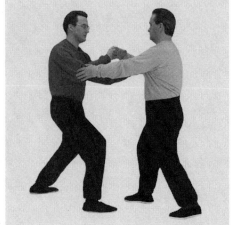

The above constitutes the *Right-Style*. The *Left-Style* is identical, only the Pushing and Neutralizing hands and the feet are reversed.

These gestures, in respect to beginners, are not to be full circular movements. You should first seek to comply with the *Four Corners*. When fully experienced with the *Four Corners*, then practice using the circular forms. In addition, you must consistently practice so that the entire body, waist and legs, every aspect will acquire externally the energies of Adhering and Sticking. This will also assist in the development of heating the kidneys, which will in turn greatly strengthen the entire spinal region.

Translator's Comments

The reference to the *Four Corners* here means "the-square-within-the-circle." This is a term that denotes both the four cardinal and diagonal directions, which are sometimes called the *Four Sides* and *Four Corners*. The point being is that in any of these exercises you would never turn from north all the way to west, rather from north to northwest or northeast, going all the way to the west or east would expose your backside, making you defective. This advice is given because beginners have a tendency to overdo the circling, thus creating defective positioning and the inability of applying efficiency to a gesture. Once you feel that your movements are precise and not exaggerated through the practice of applying the *Four Corners,* the circles will come of themselves, and they will be much more refined and exacting. Really pay attention to this, as it is the fault and downfall of many who practice *Sensing-Hands.*

The *heating of the kidneys* and *strengthening the spine* are crucial to the development of T'ai Chi skills. When the kidneys are heated they will help generate more blood flow throughout the body, thus more *Ch'i* as well. When the spine is strengthened, the *Ch'i* can flow more easily and the spirit *(Shen)* will also be strengthened.

Pushing & Warding-Off

Enclosed Stance Sequence

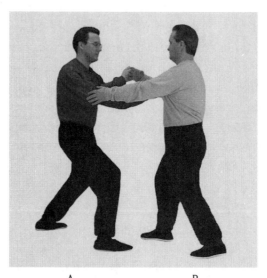

A   B

Starting Position

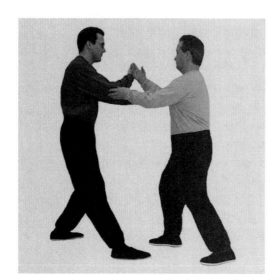
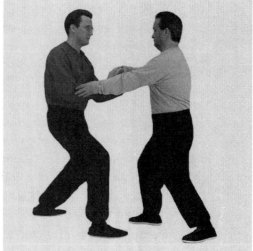

A's Enticing Circle, B's Neutralizing Circle

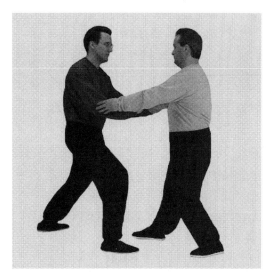
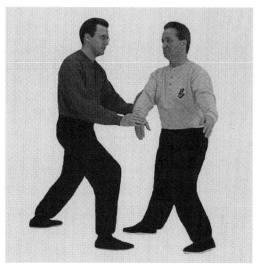

A's Pushing, B's Withdraw Neutralizing and Looking-Left

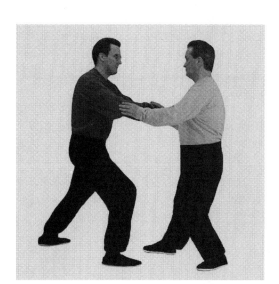
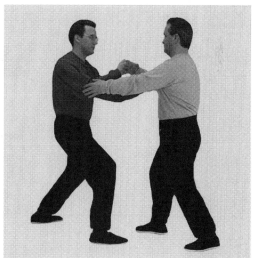

A's Looking-Left to Starting Position,
B's Gazing-Right and Advance to Starting Position

B now performs A's movements.

Third Style

Pushing & Rolling-Back

(Two-Hand, Pushing and Rolling-Back T'ui-Shou Method)

Instructions for Right-Style Training
Fixed-Stance
High Posturing, Enclosed Stance

Starting Position

Both players stand opposite of one another, each bringing their right foot forward one step. *A* places the back of his left hand onto the back of *B*'s left hand and wrist for Enticing. *A*'s right hand is on *B*'s left elbow. *A*'s Pushing gesture will be directed towards *B*'s heart.

B's left hand and arm are brought into a slightly curved position, and his right hand Adheres near *A*'s left elbow.

Both players are standing in Right-Style Bow Stances.

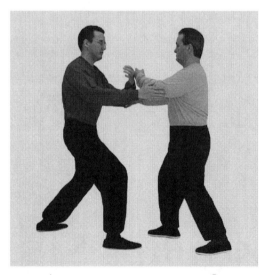

A   B

A's Enticing Circle and Pushing

A initiates his Push towards B's heart region.

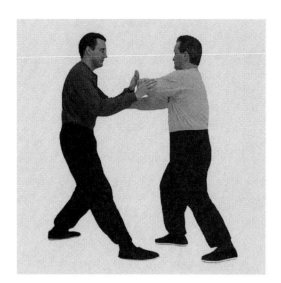

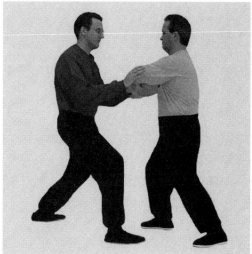

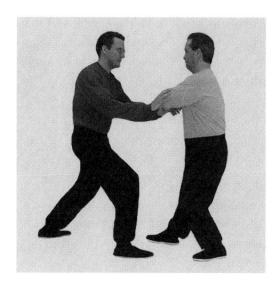

Translator's Comments

Since *A*'s left hand *Sticks* to *B*'s left hand, when *A* makes the Enticing Circle, it is the left hand which turns over and *Adheres* to *B*'s left hand. The right hand is already *Adhering* to *B*'s elbow.

B's Neutralizing Circle and Rolling-Back

To perform Neutralizing, *B* circles to the right and then shifts directly back, retaining the intent and energy of Warding-Off. *B* seats his waist, relaxes the coccyx and seats the rear leg until such time that *A*'s energy is exhausted.

When *A* Pushes, *B* uses the energy of the waist and legs to Withdraw into the rear leg, turn towards the left side, and initiate Rolling-Back. When doing so *B* brings the back of his left hand to Stick onto the back of *A*'s left-hand wrist (a seizing and turning gesture). *B*'s right hand and fore-arm Adheres along the side of *A*'s arm. *B* has performed a Rolling-Back gesture towards the left side.

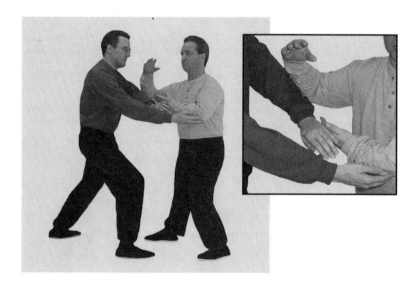

Return to Starting Position

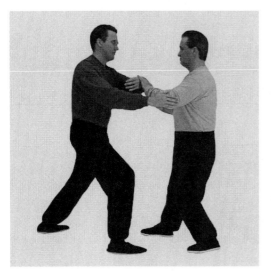 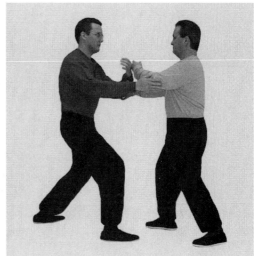

After Rolling-Back, *B* changes to do Enticing and Pushing. *A* then changes to do Neutralizing and Rolling-Back. After Rolling-Back, *A* changes to Entice and Push again.

These instructions represent the *Right-Style*. The *Left-Style* method and procedures are exactly the same, only the left foot of each player is placed in front, and the right arm is brought up into Warding-Off. It is only the hands and feet that are opposite.

THIRD STYLE
Pushing & Rolling-Back
Enclosed Stance Sequence

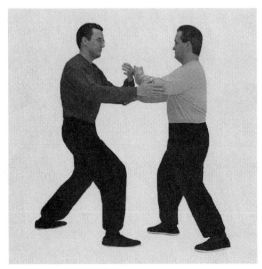

A   B

Starting Position

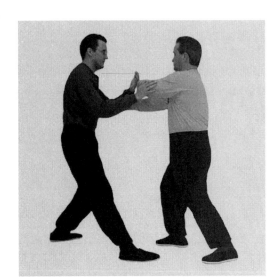

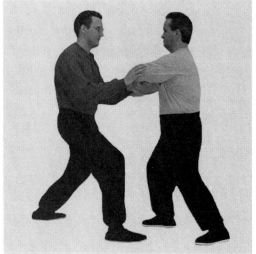

A's Enticing Circle, B's Neutralizing Circle

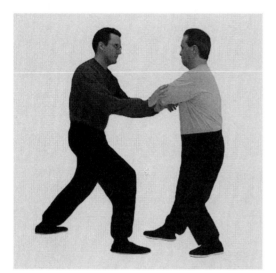
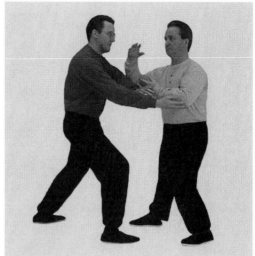

A's Pushing, B's Rolling-Back

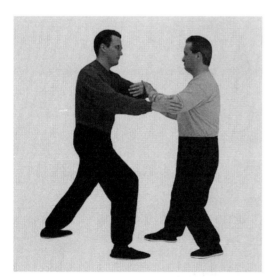
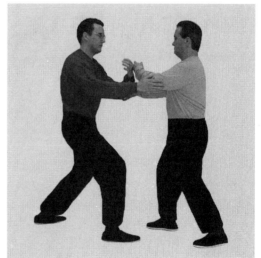

A's Looking-Left to Starting Position,
B's Gazing-Right and Advance to Starting Position

B now performs A's movements.

Pulling-Back & Neutralizing

(Two-Hand, Single Pulling-Back T'ui-Shou Method)

Instructions for Right-Style Training
Fixed-Stance
High Posturing, Enclosed Stance

Starting Position

Both players stand opposite of one another, each bringing their right foot forward one step. Both are standing in Right-Style Bow Stances.

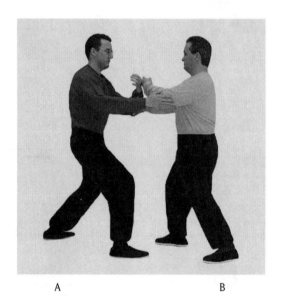

A   B

Translator's Comments

The reason why this exercise is called *Pulling-Back* instead of *Rolling-Back,* as the character *Lu* is identical with all Rolling-Back references, is that the instructions here call for *Seizing (Na)* of the opponent's left wrist. However, the Pulling-Back is done with the back of the hand—*Sticking*—while Withdrawing and turning the body. The hand turns over and the *Seizing* takes place as you drop the majority of your weight into the rear leg.

Note: The reason this exercise starts out with instructions for *B* to perform Pulling-Back is simply for the sake of showing the positioning of the hands clearly in the photographs. Although the other exercises start with *A* beginning the movements, this is irrelevant when actually practicing with a partner, as both players take turns performing each other's movements.

B's Enticing Circle and A's Neutralizing Circle

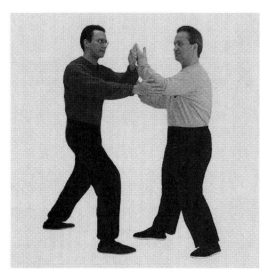 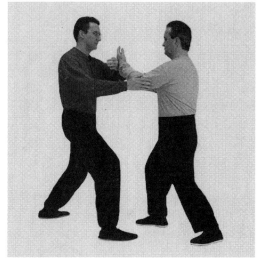

Translator's Comments

This exercise starts out the same as the others, but *B* this time performs the Enticing Circle movement. His intent, however, is to perform Pulling-Back, so he does not turn his left hand over but leaves it *Sticking* to the back of *A*'s wrist.

B's Seizing and Pulling-Back

The back of *B*'s left hand Sticks to *A*'s left hand and wrist, to make a Turning and Seizing gesture. *B*'s right forearm Adheres to the elbow of *A*'s left arm. *B* then performs Pulling-Back towards the left side.

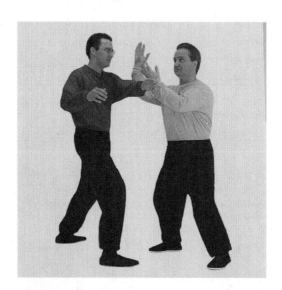

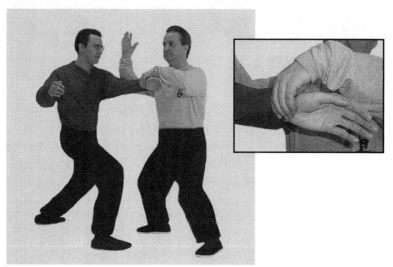

Translator's Comments

In order to perform Pulling-Back, *B* first Advances briefly into his front leg before shifting back (Withdrawing) into the rear leg again. Then, while turning his waist to the left (Looking-Left), *B Seizes* the opponent's wrist with his left hand. This *Turning and Seizing* movement is similar to Rolling-Back in how *B* attaches his right arm to *A's* left elbow. The left hand, performing the *Seizing* gesture, uses the *Crane's Beak*-type hand from *Single-Whip* posture in the T'ai Chi Ch'uan Solo Form.

When *B* performs the *Seizing* gesture to *A's* wrist, he is likewise *Adhering* to *A's* left elbow, which becomes the object of his *Issuing* (attack). Please refer to the explanation of *Neutralize, Seize,* and *Issue* in *The Intrinsic Energies of T'ai Chi Ch'uan* for more detailed information on this subject.

A's Neutralizing to Starting Position

A, having been the object of Pulling-Back, until such time that the gesture cannot proceed further, Seizes B's left wrist with his left hand by turning it up and over, and Sticks to it. The right hand and forearm Adheres to B's left arm while turning the waist. A relaxes the coccyx and seats the leg.

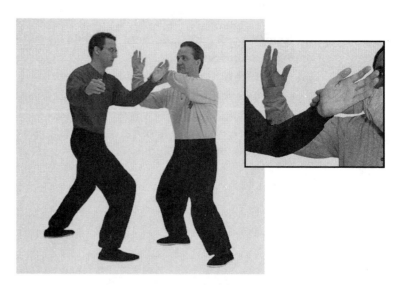

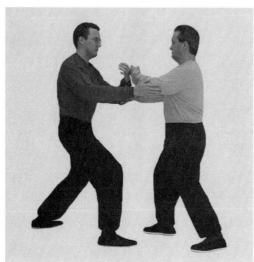

Translator's Comments

A's movements coincide with B's Enticing Circle in that he performs the Neutralizing Circle—but when B Withdraws again to perform Pulling-Back by turning the waist to the left (Looking-Left), A has to Advance and circle his waist back to the front to Neutralize in order to initiate his Enticing Circle and Pulling-Back.

When B attempts to perform Pull-Back and *Issue* to A's left elbow, A Neutralizes B's attack by first Gazing-Right, so to coincide with B's Looking-Left movement, dropping his elbow slightly and turning his waist and arm back to the left and front (Looking-Left). A's left hand is then *Sticking* to the back of B's left hand, and his right hand is *Adhering* to B's left elbow.

Changing Positions

A and B change in accordance with the movements. B is then the object of Enticing and Pulling-Back until such time that the gesture cannot proceed further. B then returns to perform Pulling-Back as in the previous instructions.

Both players follow this circling without any pause. This is the *Right-Style*. The *Left-Style* is the same except that the right and left hands are interchanged and the left foot of both players are placed in front.

FOURTH STYLE
Pulling-Back & Neutralizing
Enclosed Stance Sequence

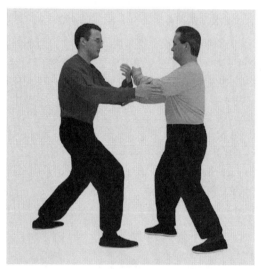

A   B

Starting Position

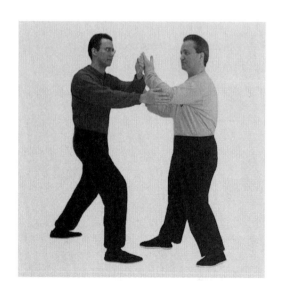
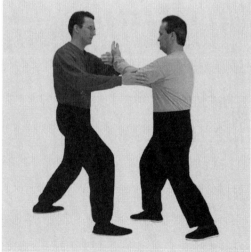

B's Enticing Circle, A's Neutralizing Circle

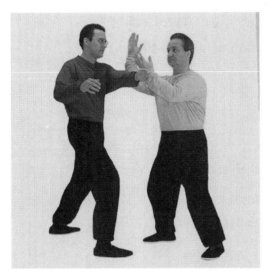
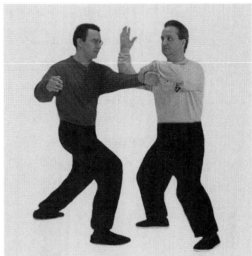

B's Seizing and Pulling-Back

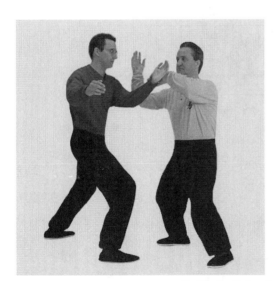
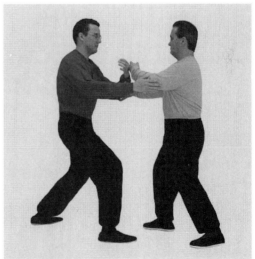

A's Neutralizing to Starting Position

A now performs B's movements.

Fifth Style

Withdraw-Pushing & Neutralizing

(Two-Hand, Pushing and Neutralizing Tui-Shou Method)

Instructions for the Right-Style Training
Fixed-Stance
High Posturing, Enclosed Stance

Starting Position

Both players stand opposite of one another, each bringing their right foot forward one step. Both players are standing in Right-Style Bow Stances.

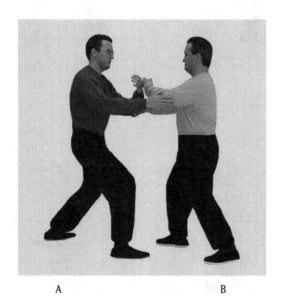

A   B

Translator's Comments

Withdraw-Pushing makes use of another variant of Neutralizing. When attaching your hand underneath to clear the opponent's hand from your elbow, there is first a Looking-Left and then a Gazing-Right movement to Neutralize. See comments under *B*'s Neutralizing Circle and Withdraw-Pushing.

A's Enticing Circle and B's Neutralizing Circle

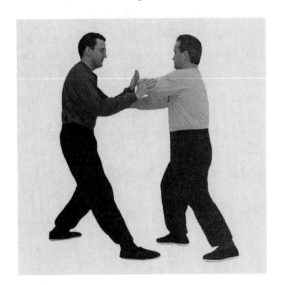 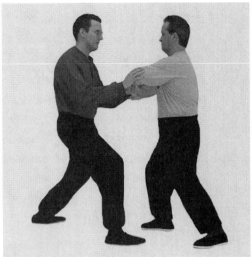

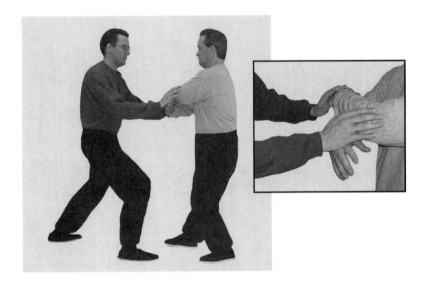

Translator's Comments

A's left hand moves from *Sticking* to *Adhering* in the same manner as in the earlier exercises.

A's Pushing and B's Withdraw-Pushing

A's left hand Adhere's to B's left wrist, and the right hand Pushes on B's left elbow. Both hands Push towards the front of B's heart region, legs ending in a Bow Stance. B seats his waist, relaxes the coccyx and seats the rear leg when Neutralizing. B Neutralizes until such time that A's Pushing energy is exhausted.

B simultaneously brings his right hand back and underneath to Stick inside of A's right hand, while using the energy of the waist and legs to turn towards the left. When readjusting his waist and legs back to face A, he turns his right hand from Sticking to Adhering and attaches his left-hand fingers onto A's right elbow.

A follows B's readjusting of the waist and legs and ends up in a Warding-Off position.

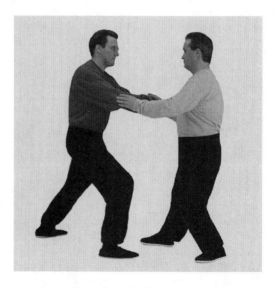

Translator's Comments

B's movements start with the Neutralizing Circle and then Withdrawing into the rear leg, where he uses a clearing gesture with his right hand to proceed into Push. This clearing gesture is identical to the action in *Withdraw-Pushing* in the T'ai Chi Solo Form. It is applied here by slightly turning the waist to the left (Looking-Left), while *Sticking* the back of the right hand behind the left arm and underneath A's right hand, which is *Adhering* to B's left elbow. The idea here is for B to wipe off the opponent's hand from his elbow. This occurs by first turning to the left and attaching the back of his right-hand fingers to *A*'s hand, and then wiping as the waist is turned back to the right and front (Gazing-Right), moving his right hand from *Sticking* to *Adhering*. When attaching the right hand to clear, it is very important not to use the wrist, but the fingers. Otherwise too much tension will be employed and the opponent will detect the intent.

Return to Starting Position—
B's Enticing Circle and Pushing,
and A's Neutralizing Circle and Withdraw-Pushing

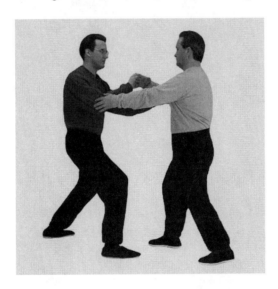

Translator's Comments

When Advancing to the Starting Position, *B* turns his right hand over to *Stick* so that he can then make the Enticing Circle and Push. The only difference is that the back of his right hand (attached to the back of *A*'s hand) moves from *Sticking* to *Adhering* when Pushing. *A*'s Withdraw-Pushing is the same as *B*'s, except that *A* clears with the left hand.

Just like above, both players—one Withdraw-Pushing and the other Neutralizing—alternate positions without pause. This is the *Right-Style*. The *Left-Style* is identical, only the right front feet are interchanged for the left. Also, while Neutralizing you must turn towards the right.

FIFTH STYLE
Withdraw-Pushing & Neutralizing
Enclosed Stance Sequence

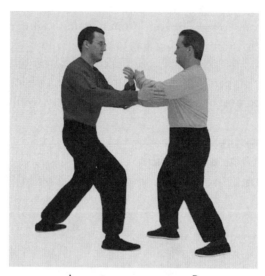

A   B

Starting Position

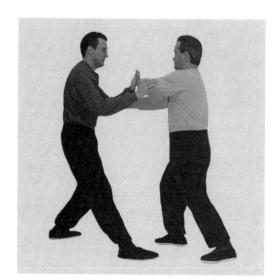

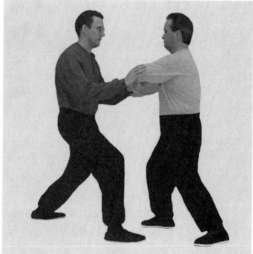

A's Enticing Circle, B's Neutralizing Circle

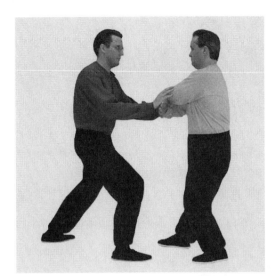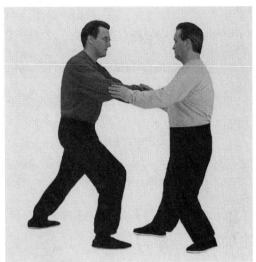

A's Pushing, B's Withdraw-Pushing

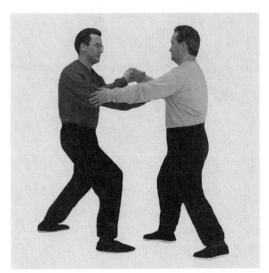

Shift to Starting Position for changing sides

B now performs A's movements.

Sixth Style

Rolling-Back & Pressing

(Two-Hand, Rolling-Back and Pressing T'ui-Shou Method)

Instructions for Right-Style Training
Fixed-Stance
High Posturing, Enclosed Stance

Starting Position

Both players stand opposite of one another, each bringing their right foot forward one step to be in Right-Style Bow Stances.

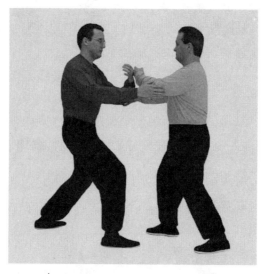

A   B

A's *Enticing Circle* and B's *Neutralizing Circle*

A initiates the movements by Enticing and Advancing to Push, and *B* performs the Neutralizing Circle before Withdrawing and Rolling-Back diagonally to the left side.

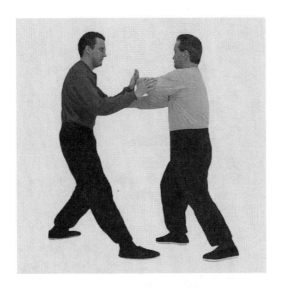

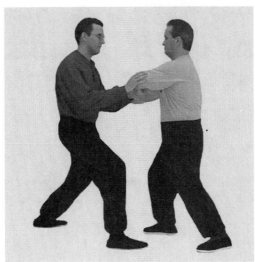

A's Pushing and B's Rolling-Back

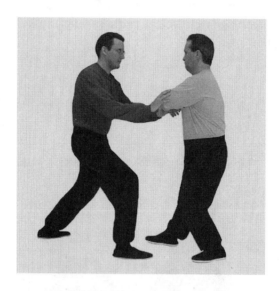

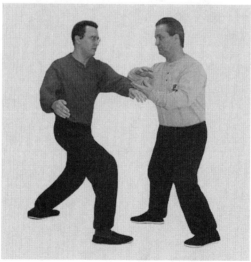

Translator's Comments
Note the position of *B*'s right arm in this Rolling-Back move-
ment, which is similar to the T'ai Chi Solo Form posture of
Wave Hands in Clouds.

A's Pressing

A, the object of Rolling-Back, avails himself of this movement by changing his left arm into a half circular shape, along with placing his right hand between the elbow and wrist (but closer to the wrist) in a Pressing position. The left arm then Presses directly towards B's chest.

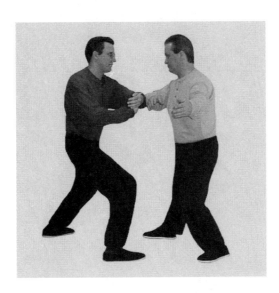

Translator's Comments

As B performs his Rolling-Back (Looking-Left) movement, A Gazes-Right and proceeds into Press by turning his waist back to the front (Looking-Left), bringing his left arm into a Warding-Off position, and attaching his right hand near to his left wrist. A then presses directly towards B's chest.

It is important that when Pressing not to sweep the left forearm across the opponent's body, as this will make your Pressing energy meaningless and ineffective. Correctly, you Press directly towards the opponent's chest. When Neutralized by the opponent, then follow the movement across (to your left).

B's Sticking and Seizing Gesture

B Neutralizes A's Press by Withdrawing into the rear leg and Seizing A's Pressing arm. He then performs Rolling-Back to the right.

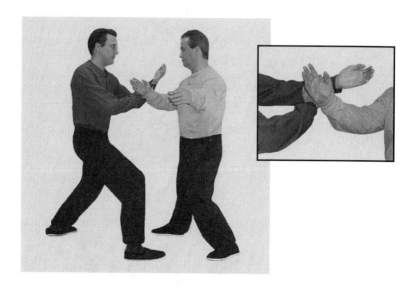

B's Rolling-Back

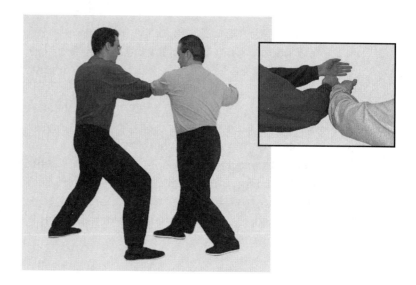

Translator's Comments

After *B* uses the Neutralizing Circle and Rolling-Back (Looking-Left) movements to Neutralize *A*'s Enticing and Pushing at the start of the exercise, he likewise adjusts his waist and legs to coincide with *A*'s movement into Press. So from his initial Roll-Back (Looking-Left), he rises in his rear leg, turns his waist back to the front (Gazing-Right), and then sinks, re-rooting into the rear leg and ending in a Warding-Off position.

As *A* then Presses forward, *B* turns his waist slightly to the right while *Sticking* and *Seizing* *A*'s Pressing hand with his right hand. *Sticking* and *Seizing* is commonly applied from a Warding-Off position in order to induce an opponent into Rolling-Back, or some other type of Neutralizing position.

In this case, *B Sticks* and *Seizes* in order to perform Rolling-Back, which he then applies to the right side (Gazing-Right). As *B* Rolls-Back, his left arm slides up along *A*'s right arm so that his left elbow attaches near *A*'s right elbow.

It is extremely important not to use the *energy of the hands and elbows* to force the Rolling-Back of the opponent to the right. Instead, *use the energy of the waist and legs* and lightly attach the right hand when *Sticking* and *Seizing,* as well as the left forearm and elbow when completing the Rolling-Back to the right.

B Sticks and *Seizes* *A*'s Pressing arm with his right hand, but he performs Rolling-Back with his left arm and elbow. He ends the movement with his left hand and forearm *Sticking* to *A*'s right hand and forearm.

B's Pressing and A's Withdraw Neutralizing

Then, in conjunction with this movement, B's right hand is then placed near his left wrist. Using the left arm, B begins Pressing towards the front of A's chest. A, when the object of Pressing, Neutralizes slightly towards his right and back. A seats his waist, relaxes the coccyx and seats the rear leg.

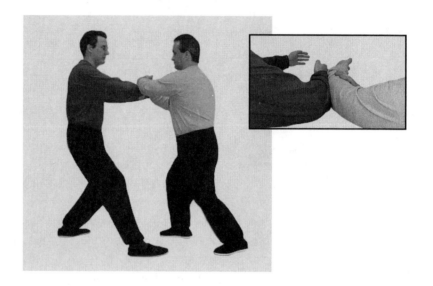

Translator's Comments

B, who is seated in his rear left leg Rolling-Back (Gazing-Right), now moves into Press by rising and turning back to the front (Looking-Left). While turning left, he puts his left arm into a Warding-Off position and attaches his right hand on his left arm to Press. He then Advances forward and Presses.

A's Sticking and Seizing Gesture

With his right hand, *A* Sticks and Seizes *B*'s left wrist. He then Adheres his left hand and forearm to *B*'s right arm and elbow while performing Rolling-Back to the right.

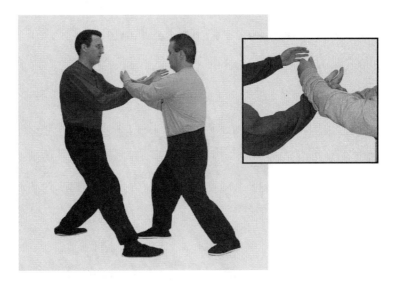

A's Rolling-Back

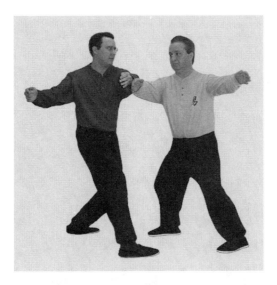

Translator's Comments
A Neutralizes B's Pressing movement by Withdrawing into the
rear leg, starting his turn to the right while *Sticking* and *Seizing*
B's Pressing hand with his right hand, and then completing his
Gazing-Right movement by Rolling-Back with his left arm.

A's Pressing and B's Withdraw Neutralizing

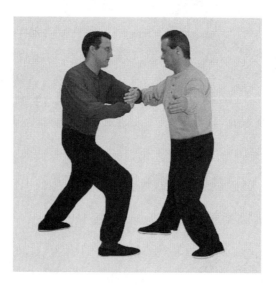

B's Sticking and Seizing Gesture

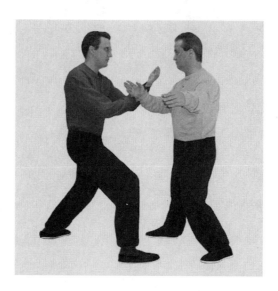

Return to Starting Position

When the movement of A's Rolling-Back is exhausted, he then proceeds into Pressing again. B then Sticks and Seizes to Neutralize A's Press and return to the starting position.

B then repeats the exercise by performing the initial Enticing and Pushing movements, and A Neutralizes and performs Rolling-Back to his left. This is the *Right-Style*. The *Left-Style* is identical, only the hands, feet, and procedures are opposite.

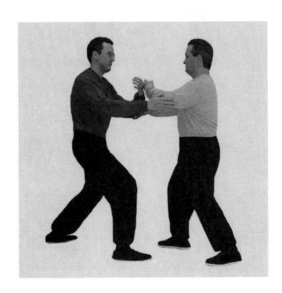

Sixth Style

Rolling-Back & Pressing

Enclosed Stance Sequence

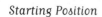

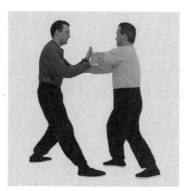

Starting Position   A's Enticing Circle, B's Neutralizing Circle

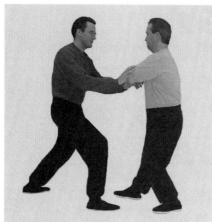

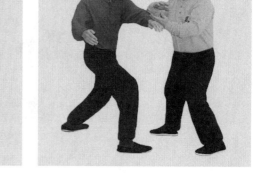

A's Pushing, B's Rolling-Back

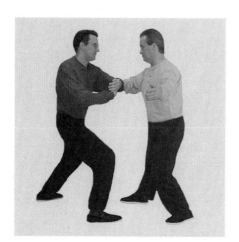

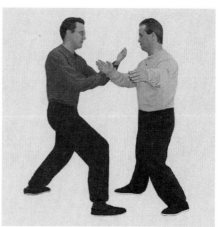

A's Pressing, B's Sticking and Seizing Gesture

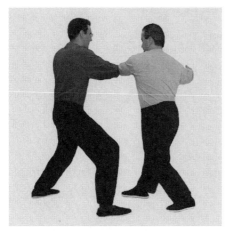

B's Rolling-Back

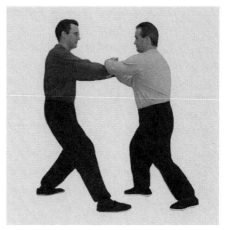

B's Pressing, A's Withdraw Neutralizing

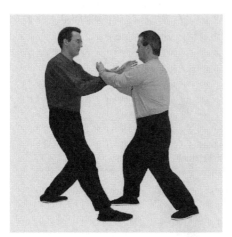

A's Sticking and Seizing Gesture

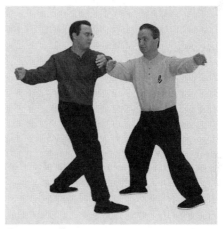

A's Rolling-Back

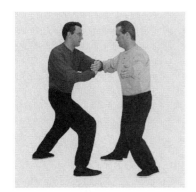

A's Pressing, B's Withdraw Neutralizing

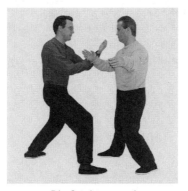

B's Sticking and
Seizing Gesture

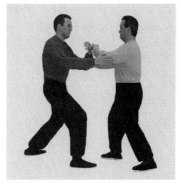

Return to Starting Position

B now performs A's movements.

Seventh Style

Thrusting & Neutralizing

(Two-Hand, Folding-Up T'ui-Shou Method)

Instructions for Right-Style Training
Fixed-Stance
High Posturing, Enclosed Stance

The actual name of this method is *Pressing the Wrist and Pushing the Elbow T'ui-Shou Method,* but since these movements are all initiated by Thrusting, it was decided to use that term.

Starting Position

Both players stand opposite of one another, each bringing their right foot forward one step, standing in Right-Style Bow Stances.

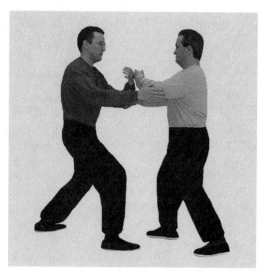

A   B

A's Enticing Circle and B's Neutralizing Circle

After A performs the Enticing Circle, he brings the back of his left hand
to Stick directly onto the back upper side of B's left wrist, with the palm
facing up and the fingers pointing directly forward. A's right hand
Adheres to B's left elbow. B is in a Warding-Off position, with his right
hand Adhering near to A's left elbow.

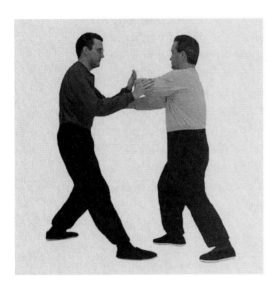
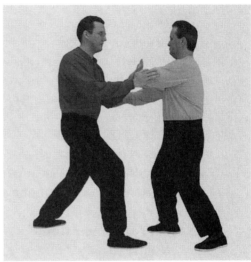

A's Thrusting and Pushing

Towards the front of B's chest, A Thrusts (Ch'a) with his left hand. The right
hand performs Pushing on B's left elbow.

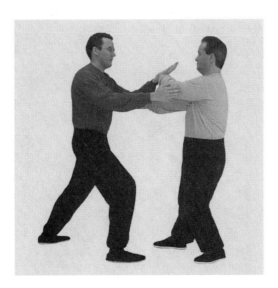

Translator's Comments

The waist and leg movements of this exercise follow the same manner as outlined in the *Fifth Style: Withdraw-Pushing & Neutralizing*. A performs the Enticing Circle and Advances to Thrust. Since A's intention is to Thrust with his left hand, however, and not Push, he leaves his hand in a *Sticking* position and does not turn it over when Enticing.

A begins the exercise *Sticking on the back upper side* of B's left wrist. Then as he Withdraws and circles to Entice, his *Sticking* hand, likewise, circles over from the wrist to the back of B's left hand and fingers—staying in its palm up position with the fingers pointing directly towards B's body.

Then as A Advances to Thrust, his right hand, which is *Adhering* to B's left elbow, Pushes the elbow down and into B's body. This Pushing movement with A's right hand acts as a lever of sorts, causing his left hand to Thrust upwards towards B's throat. (See note at the end of this exercise about how to first practice this movement.)

B's Slicing and Neutralizing

After Neutralizing A's Enticing gesture, and when the object of his Thrusting, B first shifts back to Neutralize, then avails himself of the movement by turning the waist towards the left, relaxes the coccyx and sits into the rear leg. While turning leftward, with the body upright and using the energy of the waist and legs, B drops his left elbow and Slices his hand towards A's wrist. As B turns his waist back to the front, his left hand Sticks on top of A's left wrist, with his fingers pointing towards A's heart.

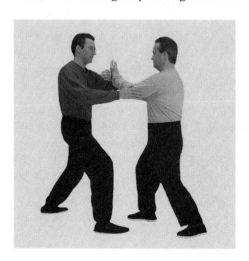

Return to Starting Position—with B then Enticing and Thrusting

B then shifts into the front leg before Withdrawing back to the rear to perform the Enticing Circle and Advance to Thrusting. His right hand performs Pushing on A's left elbow.

> #### Translator's Comments
> After performing the Neutralizing Circle, B Withdraws to his back leg, and when A Pushes down on his left elbow, B follows A's Push by dropping his left elbow and turning his waist slightly to the left (Looking-Left). As B drops his elbow and Looks-Left, he performs a *Slicing* movement with the back edge of his left hand. Meaning, B slides the edge of his left hand down the back of A's Thrusting hand to *Stick* onto A's wrist. This *Slicing* movement helps him to Neutralize A's Thrust because it enhances his ability to turn A's arm over and to the left (Looking-Left), and when B turns his waist back to the front (Gazing-Right), the *Slicing* movement enables his left hand to be *Sticking on the back upper side* of A's left wrist. B then shifts forward to be in the Starting Position and perform A's movements.

Both players Advance and Withdraw, Thrust and Neutralize, so that each are able to alternately train the movements. This is the *Right-Style*. The *Left-Style* is the same, only the hands and circling gestures are opposite. When beginning to learn this exercise, it is well advised to just use one hand at first, as it will be difficult enough just learning the practice of controlling during all the wrist movements (in method this is same as in the above description of the exercise), and in comparison is much easier.

> #### Translator's Comments
> What is being said here is that at first you should concentrate more on just keeping everything in order, which is the meaning of *"controlling,"* and not worry initially so much about Thrusting and incorporating the more advanced techniques of Folding-Up—that is, the Pushing movement when Thrusting, and the *Slicing* movement when Neutralizing.
>
> It will suffice for beginners to just perform the movements without putting too much emphasis on actually Thrusting.

Thrusting & Neutralizing

Enclosed Stance

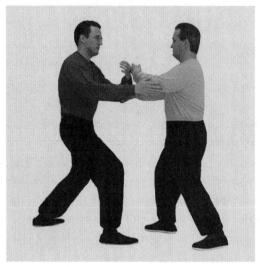

A   B

Starting Position

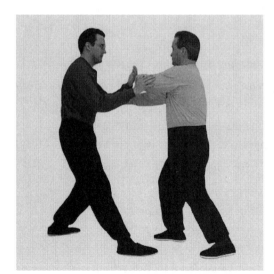
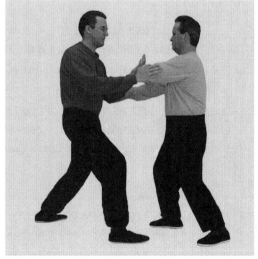

A's Enticing Circle, B's Neutralizing Circle

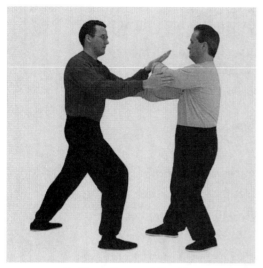

A's Thrusting and Pushing

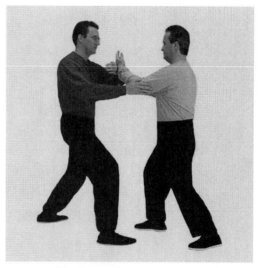

B's Slicing and Neutralizing

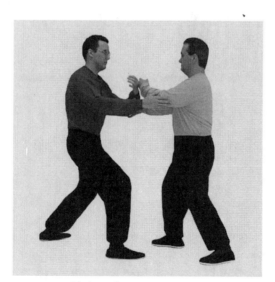

Shift to Starting Position

B now performs A's movements.

Single-Hand Circular-Thrusting

(Single-Hand, Standing Circular T'ui-Shou Method)

Instructions for Right-Style Training
Fixed-Stance
High Posturing, Enclosed Stance

Starting Position

Both players stand in opposite Bow Stances of one another, each bringing their right foot forward one step. *B* places the edge of his right-
hand palm directly unto *A*'s upper right-hand wrist.

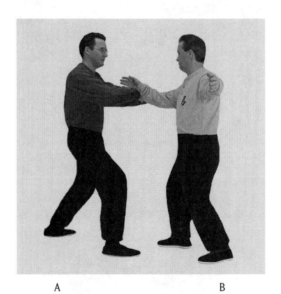

A   B

Translator's Comments

A is in a Warding-Off position with his right arm in a half circular shape. In this exercise, as in the First Style, only one
arm is being practiced. *A* and *B*'s left arms are extended outwards with the palms facing forward.

B's Slicing and A's Warding-Off Circle

Using the energy of the waist and legs, towards the rear and moving downward, B circles as though Slicing (Chieh) A's right hand.

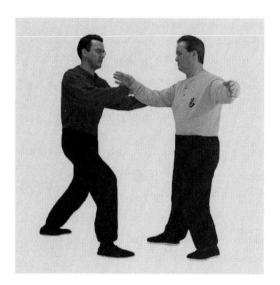
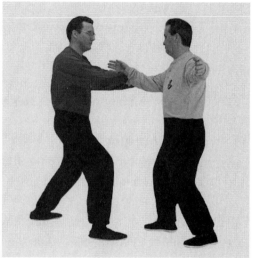

B's Thrusting to A's Abdomen

Immediately following his Slicing movement, B Thrusts towards A's abdomen.

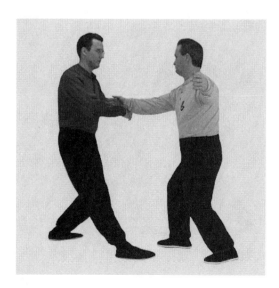

Translator's Comments

When *B* performs Thrusting, his right hand stays in the
Thrusting position and does not turn over as he makes the initial, standard Enticing-Circle movements of his waist and legs.
With the edge of his Thrusting hand, however, *A* parallels the
movements of his waist and legs by also making a circling—
Slicing—gesture along the opponent's wrist. This is just a
small circle and should not be applied with force or tension.

Compare the differences in the Thrusting movements of
this exercise with the *Seventh Style: Thrusting & Neutralizing.*

A's Neutralizing

With *A*'s right arm in a Warding-Off position, *A* first Neutralizes *B*'s Enticing
movement and then avails himself of *B*'s incoming Thrust by seating his
waist, relaxing the coccyx and Withdrawing into his rear leg. After this
movement of going back and downwards, *A* continues Neutralizing by
turning to the right side. When the Neutralizing has reached the right side
of *A*'s rib area, he begins to rise into an upright stance with the right arm
in a half circular shape, positioning his two hands into a shape of a partial
circle and line (like a bow and its string), raising them upwards until reaching levelly alongside his right ear.

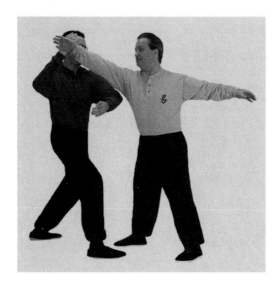

Translator's Comments

A Neutralizes first through the Neutralizing Circle and the Withdrawing movement to the rear leg. He then turns his waist to the right (Gazing-Right), and rises into an upright position. His arms, maintaining their Warding-Off positions, follow this rising gesture until his right hand draws up alongside his right ear, and the left hand, held out in a ready position, hovers underneath the opponent's right elbow. It is this position of his hands and arms that looks as if he is holding and drawing a Bow.

A's Enticing and Thrusting to B's Forehead

A then extends out his right arm bringing the fingers to perform Thrusting to B's forehead. When performing this there is first a half circling gesture of the upper right hand, and the body should be standing upright while circling.

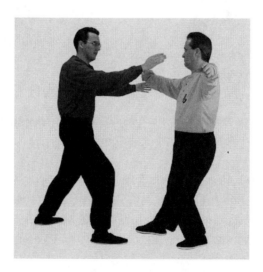

Translator's Comments

This half circling gesture is meant to be a small circling gesture that draws in the opponent's energy (Enticing) and upsets his center of balance. This movement, which starts in the rear leg from the Gazing-Right position, allows A to adjust his waist and legs back to the front (Looking-Left), before he Advances and Thrusts to B's forehead.

B's Neutralizing

B, availing himself of A's incoming gesture, Neutralizes by bringing his arm into a bent bow shape [Warding-Off] and Withdrawing into the rear leg, seating his waist and relaxing the coccyx. He then brings A's hand up and out to Entice. The right hand Sticks to B's wrist.

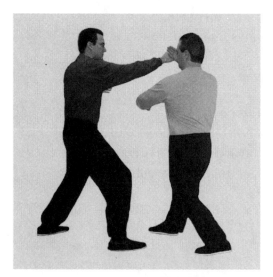 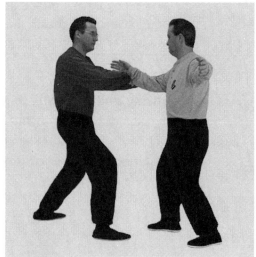

Starting Position

After moving back and down, B Entices by performing Slicing to A's hand and wrist, and then Thrusts to B's abdomen.

Both players repeat this pattern of exercise. The movements of A are similar to the *Step Back to Chase the Monkey Away* T'ai Chi Ch'uan Solo Form posture. B's are like the *Squatting Downward* Solo Form posture. The *Left-Style* training is identical, only the left feet step to the front, and the left arms Circle and Thrust.

Translator's Comments

The reader should note that this is the only exercise which does not automatically alternate sides. B performs Enticing and Thrusting at abdomen level in a slight squatting position, and A performs Enticing and Thrusting at head level. They can practice in this manner indefinitely; however, to change positions A initiates the following movements.

Changing Positions—A's Slicing and Thrusting to B's Abdomen

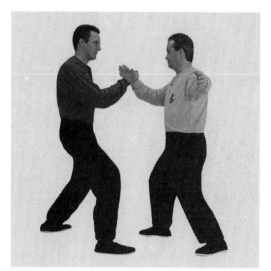 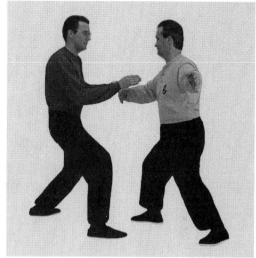

Translator's Comments

After *B* performs Enticing to the right to lead into Thrusting to *A*'s abdomen again, *A* circumvents *B*'s Thrust by performing Enticing himself. In this case, when *B* Advances to the front to perform his Thrust, *A* drops his right elbow while slightly turning his waist to the right (Gazing-Right) and *Slicing* his right hand up to *B*'s wrist, before turning his waist back to the front (Looking-Left). *B*'s arm turns over into a Warding-Off position. *A* then Withdraws into the rear leg to perform the Slicing and Thrusting movements to *B*'s abdomen.

   Thrusting is a rare technique of Sensing-Hands, and is usually not associated or discussed within popular books on T'ai Chi Ch'uan. It is essential, however, to train it and understand its importance. On a brutal level *Thrusting* is used to jab the eyes or solar plexus in a whip-like fashion. On a much more refined level it is used for closing off *ch'i* cavities. There are thirty-six such cavities in the human body which can be fatal, and seven that are fatal. *Thrusting* is the initial training method for what is called *Closing Ch'i Cavities.*

   Slicing is a means by which to initiate *Enticing* energy. It is also means to initially *Seize,* the method of obstructing the *Ch'i* meridians in the body.

EIGHTH STYLE
Single-Hand, Circular-Thrusting
Enclosed Stance Sequence

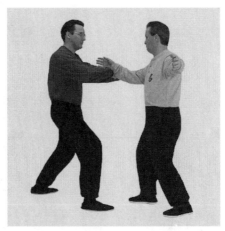

Starting Position

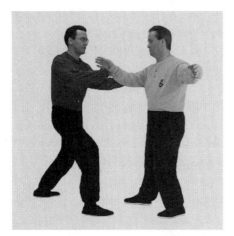
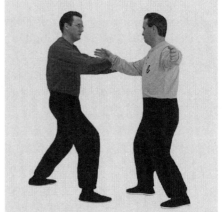

B's Slicing, A's Warding-Off Circle

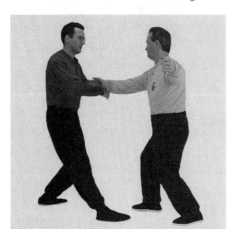
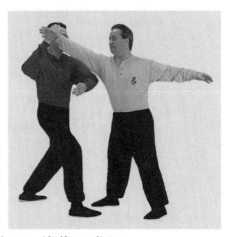

B's Thrusting to A's Abdomen, A's Neutralizing

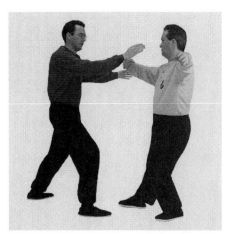
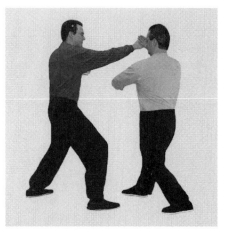

A's Enticing and Thrusting to B's Forehead, B's Neutralizing

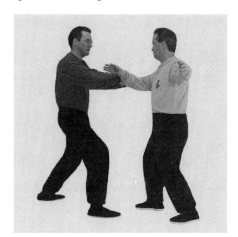

Return to Starting Position

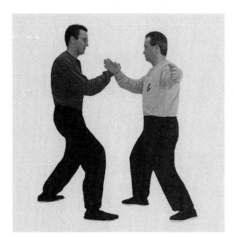
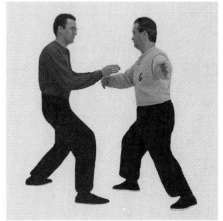

Changing Position
(A turns B's arm over to perform the Slicing and Enticing Circle, then Thrusts to B's abdomen)

The Four Skills
of Sensing-Hands

(Fixed-Stance and Active-Steps Styles)

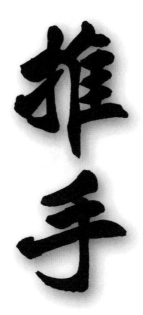

An Explanation of Adhering, Sticking, Joining, and Following—and Opposing, Leaning, Discarding, and Resisting

After training to an appropriate stage with the practice of T'ai Chi Ch'uan, there are those who anxiously desire to achieve higher skills and acquire complete explanations as to what is meant by *Adhering, Sticking, Joining, and Following,* and their defective counterparts of *Opposing, Leaning, Discarding, and Resisting.*

Translator's Comments

An appropriate stage is having acquired some Root (Fixed-Rooting), the sensation of *Ch'i* in the *Tan-T'ien,* ability to apply the Mind-Intent *(Yi)* to your movements, a degree of skill in applying the principles of T'ai Chi Ch'uan, and the ability to move the body as a whole unit. All this can be gained from just the practice of the T'ai Chi Ch'uan Solo Form. Next, there should be a degree of skill in the practices of Sensing-Hands. When an *appropriate stage* is acquired, the following discourse will make sense to the practitioner. As you progress, more and more of it will become apparent to you about the profoundness of this subject.

As separate words, some people may have knowledge of these, yet the meanings are unclear to them in relation to *Sensing-Hands.* Some are aware of these names, yet do not understand what the true meanings are. So they desire the ability to grasp the meanings of these eight words—one by one distinguishing clearly all the particulars associated to them. But these meanings, in their highest sense, are like the horn of a unicorn, the scales of a dragon, or the feathers of a phoenix, if too much is seen of them it would be unbearable.

Translator's Comments

These things are considered so rare and exceptional for a human being to see that the mind cannot grasp or take in the splendor, and so it is an unbearable experience for human eyes.

Notwithstanding, if these eight words are unclear you will be incapable of acquiring *Interpreting Energy* (*Tung Chin*). If you do not acquire *Interpreting Energy*, in the end you will have entirely lost the efficacy of the practical use of *Sensing-Hands*.

The old, original writings on T'ai Chi Ch'uan say nothing in regards to the *Four Skills of Sensing-Hands in Fixed-Stance* methods of Warding-Off, Rolling-Back, Pressing, and Pushing. But they do discuss these eight words—*Adhering, Sticking, Joining, Following, Opposing, Leaning, Discarding,* and *Resisting*—so we must then first examine their meanings. Analyzing them in detail one by one, so that those who are learning may apprehend the underlying principles of these writings. Afterwards it will be easier to progress, and to forego the corrupted practice of forsaking the essentials and following the inferior.

Translator's Comments

See the Preface under *About the Translation* for my comments on the "old and original" teachings.

In the *T'ai Chi Ch'uan Treatise* there is a closing verse in which the *Eight Postures* are mentioned in association with the *Eight Diagrams* of the *Book of Changes,* as well as with the *Eight Directions.* However, this verse is an obvious addition to the classic as it does not follow the same rhythm or even theme of the earlier text. Other than the addition mentioned above, there is no mention of the four terms of Warding-Off, Rolling-Back, Pressing, and Pushing. However, there are many references to *Adhering, Sticking, Joining,* and *Following.*

More probable is that Chen is referring to even earlier works that deal with the subject of T'ai Chi Boxing. For an excellent overview of the more plausible origins of T'ai Chi and related writings of earlier masters, I refer the reader to *Lost T'ai-chi Classics from the Ch'ing Dynasty* by Douglas

Wile and to *Chinese Boxing—Masters and Methods* by Robert W. Smith. In the appendix section of Smith's book, see *Chou Chi-Ch'un's Views on the Origin of T'ai Chi.*

Adhering *(Chan)* means to raise the opponent upwards so he can be uprooted. This is called *Kao* (correctly causing the opponent to float).

Translator's Comments
This is the correct intent and energy of Warding-Off.

Sticking *(Nien)* means to prevent the opponent from being able to separate from you. This is called *Ch'uan* (correctly attaching to the opponent).

Translator's Comments
This is the correct intent and energy of Rolling-Back.

Joining *(Lien)* means to give yourself up to the opponent's movement. This is called *Wu Li* (correctly not separating from the opponent).

Translator's Comments
This is the correct intent and energy of Pressing.

Following *(Sui)* means that when the opponent moves you must move. This is called *Ying* (correctly adapting to the opponent's changes).

Translator's Comments
This is the correct intent and energy of Pushing.

These four words are the primary foundation and essential guidelines of T'ai Chi Ch'uan. Without them, it would be as if there were no spirit or wisdom incorporated to your practice. It takes vigorous effort in order to comprehend the meaning of these words. If you are incapable of *Interpreting*, then as a student you must seek to learn it. In addition, you must give great attention to these following four words as well.

Opposing *(Ting)*, which is called *Chu Tou* (wrongly confronting the opponent).

Translator's Comments
This is the defective application of Warding-Off.

Leaning *(Pien)*, which is called *Pu Chi* (wrongly avoiding the opponent).

Translator's Comments
This is the defective application of Rolling-Back.

Discarding *(Tiu)*, which is called *Li Kai* (wrongly separating from the opponent).

Translator's Comments
This is the defective application of Pressing.

Resisting *(Kang)*, which is called *T'ai Kuo* (wrongly giving too much energy to the opponent).

Translator's Comments
This is the defective application of Pushing.

These four words when held in comparison with *Adhering, Sticking, Joining,* and *Following*, are their defective counterparts. If there is *Opposing, Leaning, Discarding,* and *Resisting*, the end result is that you will be unable to bring about *Adhering, Sticking, Joining,* and *Following*. In contradistinction, if you have the abilities of *Adhering, Sticking, Joining,* and *Following*, you will certainly be devoid of the corruption's of *Opposing, Leaning, Discarding,* and *Resisting*. So when you begin learning *Sensing-Hands*, each of these four words can easily transgress themselves into a corruption or defect.

The Four Skills of Sensing-Hands in Fixed-Stance

Warding-Off, Rolling-Back, Pressing, and Pushing

The very foundation for acquiring the skills *(Kung Fu)* of T'ai Chi Ch'uan rests entirely with your ability to *Interpret (Tung Chin)*. Yet, it is impractical to seek after *Interpreting Energy* without first acquiring *Adhering, Sticking, Joining,* and *Following*. Even if you sought to just acquire the two basic energies of *Adhering* and *Sticking (Chan Nien Chin)*, without first training *Fixed-Stance Sensing-Hands*, it would be really quite impractical and pointless.

Fixed-Stance Sensing-Hands has the divisions of *Enclosed Stances (Ho Pu)* and *Direct Stances (Shun Pu)*. The *Enclosed Stances* of *Sensing-Hands* are the procedure whereby both persons each step out in an identical manner. For example, *A* would bring forward the right foot, and *B* would likewise do the same. Then both persons, with both hands joined, turn and circle in the prescribed directions, moving from either an upright position *(Cheng)* or from a low, seated position *(Tao)*—these movements are also called *Shun* (Staying and Going With) and *Yao* (Twisting and Breaking Off), and each are very practical and useful.

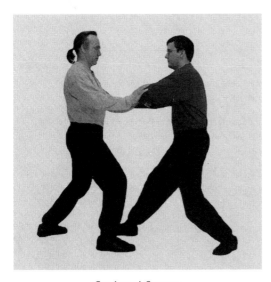

Enclosed Stance

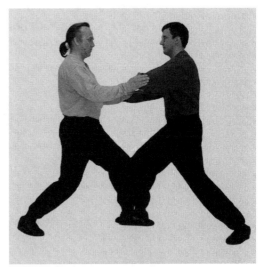

Direct Stance

Translator's Comments

When both players stand in Bow Stances with the same leg forward, it is called *Enclosed Stance* because the feet create an image of allowing nothing to be able to enter on either side.

The terms *Cheng* and *Tao* need some explanation as they are not commonly referred to in T'ai Chi Ch'uan manuals. *Cheng* positioning is where both players stand joined together and make use of turning, rising, and sinking, shifting forwards and backwards. The movements of *Cheng* require staying attached and going with the movements of each player, with no drastic changes in either the height or circumference of the posturing. These movements are what is normally seen and practiced in mainstream Sensing-Hands training. *Cheng* movements are also sometimes referred to as *Shun* (Staying and Going With) movements.

Tao movements are very different than those of *Cheng*. *Tao* movements are much more advanced and require low dropping down and high upright rising gesturing, twisting and breaking away movements, with constant drastic changes in both the height and circumference of the movements. *Tao* movements are then sometimes referred to as *Yao* (Twisting and Breaking Away) movements.

Direct Stances of Sensing-Hands are consequently just the opposite. If A steps forward with the left foot, B will then step forward with the right foot, and vice versa. Then with both their hands they turn and circle in the prescribed directions. With *Direct Stances* it is enough to just perform the *Cheng* posturing—*Shun* (Staying and Going With) movements.

Translator's Comments

The *Direct Stances* are so-named because the opposite legs of each player are placed directly and closely together.

The positioning of either *Cheng* or *Tao* can be performed in either Enclosed Stances or Direct Stances, however, the text states that when performing *Direct Stances Sensing-Hands* it is enough to just perform the *Cheng* posturing. This is advised because performing the *Tao* movements within Direct Stances can become very tense and overly active by those not highly skilled in Sensing-Hands. *Tao* movements are much easier, but by no means void of difficulty, in Enclosed Stances position.

The practices of *Fixed-Stance Sensing-Hands* in former times brought about many new adaptations to later generations. After the Yang family T'ai Chi Ch'uan teachings had reached the south, the disciples there were transmitted only the methods of *Enclosed Stances of Sensing-Hands*. This caused many people to be misled about the *Direct Stances of Sensing-Hands*, as they were never told that the original practices were the *Direct Stances*, not *Enclosed Stances*.

Translator's Comments

By the *south* is meant that either Yang Cheng-fu or Chen Wei-Ming (his disciple) traveled to southern China to teach, and apparently only taught the *Enclosed Stances of Sensing-Hands* to his disciples there. Chen, in his book, claims he was the first Yang Family-style teacher to teach in the south. Others say it was Cheng-fu.

However, the *Enclosed Stances* and *Direct Stances* each have profitable aspects, and it is impracticable to be biased towards either one. Therefore, students should not discriminate them by solely practicing one or the other. Otherwise, if you only practice the *Enclosed Stances*, and if you happen to meet with an opponent who has also trained the *Direct Stances*, then there will be the danger of your having no way in which to adapt to the situation.

But it really does not matter when doing *Sensing-Hands* whether *Enclosed Stances* or *Direct Stances* are practiced, as long as the *Four Skills* of Warding-Off, Rolling-Back, Pressing, and Pushing are all, one by one, clearly distinguished. Beginning students must learn how to adapt to the turning and circling gestures within all the basic methods provided here, and then they will surely become considerably more adept. But without the *Four Skills* of Warding-Off, Rolling-Back, Pressing, and Pushing, and a detailed and clear analysis of their own progress, they will find it impossible to acquire the skills of *Neutralizing* and *Issuing*.

It must be understood though that it is hardly enough to just make turns and circles when engaged in *Sensing-Hands,* for in the end you will completely lose the correct principles of Warding-Off, Rolling-Back, Pressing, and Pushing. If you do not correctly know the *Four Skills,* you will then be unable to even speak about *Sensing-Hands.* For if you cannot do *Sensing-Hands* correctly, how could you ever hope to advance or find any satisfaction in your T'ai Chi Ch'uan practice?

It can be further stated that the *Four Skills* are absolutely central to *Sensing-Hands,* just as the five vowels of *a, e, i, o, u* are central to the English language. If English did not have these syllables, how could the sounds for speech be produced? This is also true of *Sensing-Hands.* If devoid of the *Four Skills,* and you sought to string together the movements uninterruptedly (like syllables strung together to make words), how could you make it happen?

The old masters discovered that Warding-Off, Rolling-Back, Pressing, and Pushing within the *Fixed-Stances* had a very high meaning, and in practice were very abstruse and profound. In the separation of one skill from another each are capable of reciprocally producing or destroying the other, identical to the Five Elements.

Contained within the Five Elements (*Wu Hsing*) are *Metal (Chin), Wood (Mu), Water (Shui), Fire (Huo),* and *Earth (Tu).* These are also called, within T'ai Chi Ch'uan, the *Five Activities,* which are *Advancing (Chien Chin), Withdrawing (Hou Tui), Looking-Left (Tso Kuan), Gazing-Right (Yu Pang),* and *Fixed-Rooting (Chung Ting).*

Advancing is represented by Metal, Withdrawing by Wood, Looking-Left by Water, Gazing-Right by Fire, and Fixed-Rooting by Earth. But you only need to classify these by Metal, Wood, Water, Fire, and Earth, as there is no need for students to examine these correlations too deeply.

But it is necessary to give full attention to the details and particulars concerning the associated movements and applications to Advancing, Withdrawing, etc., and how they apply to practical use.

In addition, beyond Warding-Off, Rolling-Back, Pressing, and Pushing there must be added the term of Neutralizing. If not, it will be impossible to string together the other four movements. In application, Neutralizing looks like Warding-Off.

Translator's Comments

In the *Four Skills of Sensing-Hands in Fixed-Stance* method to follow there are three variations of Neutralizing which connect the four movements together. These are as follows:

1) *Warding-Off Circle Neutralizing:* This is the same Neutralizing Circle movement as in all the *Eight Styles.* It is performed to counter the opponent's Enticing Circle.

2) *Gazing-Right Neutralizing:* When Press is about to be initiated, Neutralize with a slight Gazing-Right movement. The hands of the person Neutralizing *Adhere* near the elbows of the person who is Pressing. While still in the forward leg, when the opponent starts his Press, Neutralize by rising in the forward leg (Advancing) and turning slightly to the right corner (Gazing-Right). The right hand is placed slightly underneath the opponent's left elbow. When rising and turning right, lift the opponent's elbow slightly to raise his center.

3) *Looking-Left Neutralizing and Warding-Off:* From the previous Neutralize, continue circling to Neutralize by making a Withdrawing and Looking-Left movement. While turning and sinking into the rear leg, circle the left arm down and then brings it upwards into a Warding-Off position while Advancing back into the front leg.

Withdrawing is not necessarily just a Neutralizing movement. Withdrawing is primarily the method, or connecting movement, used to induce any of the *Six Energies* of *Adhering, Sticking, Neutralizing, Seizing, Enticing,* and *Issuing.*

Methods of the Four Skills in Fixed-Stance

Instructions for Right Style-Training
Fixed-Stance
High Posturing, Enclosed Stance

Starting Position

Both persons stand opposite of one another, each bringing their right foot forward one step and planting the feet. They are in Right-Style Bow Stances.

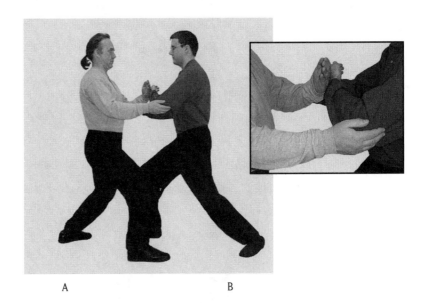

A   B

Translator's Comments

This is the same starting position as in the Eight Styles, wherein *A* and *B* are *Sticking* to the backs of each other's left hands, mutually Warding-Off.

A's Enticing Circle and B's Warding-Off Circle

A performs the Enticing Circle to lead into Push, and B, using the energy of the waist and legs, Neutralizes by bringing his left forearm slightly upwards to perform a Warding-Off circle, which retards the incoming gesture of A and completes the Warding-Off gesture.

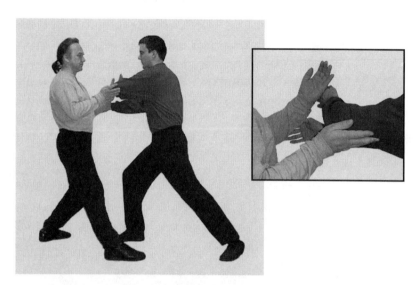

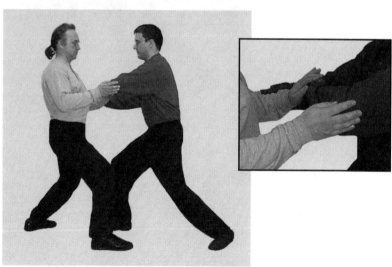

A's Pushing and B's Rolling-Back

After Enticing, A performs a double-handed Push on B's left forearm. B then Withdraws and performs Rolling-Back by making use of the momentum of the Warding-Off gesture. With the left hand and forearm (nearer the wrist area), B applies Sticking to A's left hand and forearm, and the right elbow Adheres near A's left elbow. Using the energy of the waist and legs, B turns towards the left corner into Rolling-Back. This then is the Rolling-Back gesture, with performing Looking-Left.

Neutralizing, such as in Rolling-Back and in other Looking-Left and Gazing-Right movements, is usually used to make the opponent careless about their gazing and to create the opportunity of getting the opponent to expose his backside.

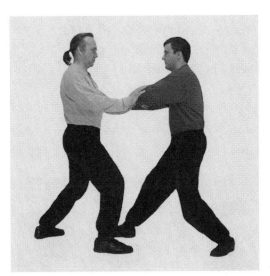 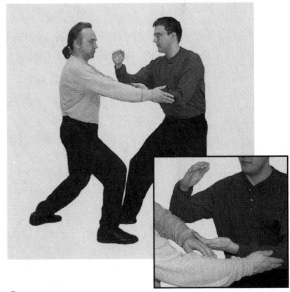

Translator's Comments

Beginners at Sensing-Hands are instructed to perform double-handed Pushing because it will be too difficult to clearly distinguish the substantial and insubstantial in an opponent, and their skills of *Interpreting* will not yet be sufficient. But as your skills grow you should be performing just a one-handed Push. In the instructions above it would be the left hand which *Issues* the Push so that it comes off the (left) rear foot. The three main reasons for becoming competent in one-handed Pushing are as follows:

1) T'ai Chi is based on *Yin* and *Yang*, both hands cannot be *Yang*, one must be held in reserve in the event the opponent makes a sudden change. In which case, the other hand would Push.

2) One hand must perform *Adhering* and the other *Sticking*, so that the opponent can either be *Issued* to or *Seized and Neutralized* instantly depending on his movements.

3) A double-handed Push can create the defect of *double-weighting*.

B's Pressing and A's Gazing-Right Neutralizing

After *B* performs Rolling-Back and begins changing his right forearm and left hand to do Pressing, *A* changes his hands to perform Gazing-Right Neutralizing.

The procedures for this Neutralizing are as follows: *A*'s left hand attaches to *B*'s right elbow, and *A*'s right hand slides down and slightly underneath *B*'s left elbow. Using the energy of the waist and legs, and the methods of hollow the chest and raise the back, *A* Advances and turns towards the right side to Neutralize.

When *B* begins Pressing, he must not allow his two arms to follow the gesturing of *A*'s Neutralizing too far to his left.

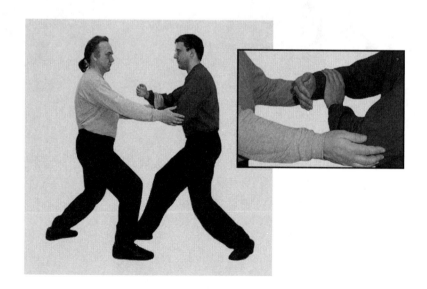

Translator's Comments

Gazing-Right Neutralizing is a subtle movement in that *A* maintains contact with *B*'s left elbow with his right hand at the conclusion of *B*'s Rolling-Back. Just as *B* is beginning to change into a Pressing gesture, *A* slides the right hand slightly underneath *B*'s left elbow and makes a slight rising and turning movement to the right (Advancing and Gazing-Right) that will cause *B* to turn out, thus disrupting his Pressing. This movement also creates the momentum for *A*'s *Looking-Left Neutralizing and Warding-Off.*

When *B* is changing from Rolling-Back into Pressing, he initially brings his right forearm down in front of the solar plexus, in a half circular shape, and brings his left hand to attach to his inner right forearm, at which time he is directly facing *A* with the weight in his rear leg.

He will then begin shifting forward (Advancing) to perform Pressing to *A*'s chest.

"When B begins Pressing, he must not allow his arms to follow the gesturing of A's Neutralizing too far to his left." This last sentence, referring to *A*'s Gazing-Right Neutralizing movement, warns *B* not to move too far left (following the Neutralize) or he will open up his back for attack. (See the comment about Neutralizing in the second paragraph under the instructions for *B*'s Rolling-Back.)

When *A* is Neutralizing, whether it be Gazing-Right or Looking-Left, it is important to train the skill of just lightly attaching the fingertips of the hands to *B*'s elbows. Then use the energy of the waist and legs to rise, turn, and sink to perform Neutralizing.

Notice that it says "lightly attach the fingertips," nowhere does it imply using forcible strength in the hands and arms. Doing so will cause several problems. The two main ones being that you give the opponent the ability to detect your intentions, and the other is that in applying force to your own hands and arms you destroy your ability to *Interpret*—which is to sense the actions and intentions of the opponent.

A's Looking-Left Neutralizing and Warding-Off, and B's Circling to Stick and Adhere

A, after Neutralizing to the right, Withdraws into the rear leg and turns the waist to the left and then back to the front [Looking-Left Neutralizing]. He then brings his left forearm upwards to perform Warding-Off, and then Advances back into the forward leg. This then is the Looking-Left Neutralizing gesture and Warding-Off, which works in conjunction with and follows his Gazing-Right gesture.

B, from his hands in the Pressing position, and following A's Neutralizing movements, circles his waist and hands out to the right and then brings them back to Stick and Adhere to A's left hand and elbow, which has ended up in Warding-Off. Both are now back in the starting position, and B then performs the Enticing Circle and Advance to Push.

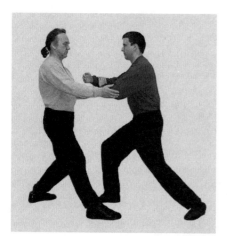
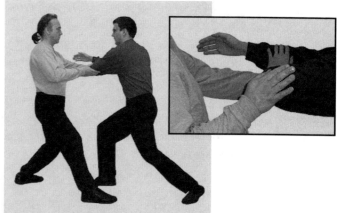

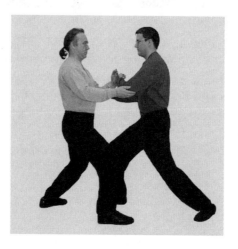

Translator's Comments

After Advancing into his forward leg and being Neutralized, *B,* whose hands are in a Pressing position, turns his waist and circles his hands up to the right (Gazing-Right) and then back and to the front (Looking-Left), attaching them to *A's* left hand and elbow. *B's* left hand *Sticks* to *A's* left hand, and his right *Adheres* near to *A's* left elbow. *B* remains in his forward leg.

A and *B* have now switched roles, with *B* now in the starting position to perform the Enticing Circle before Pushing, and *A* to perform the Warding-Off Circle before Withdrawing and then Rolling-Back.

The following instructions are recaps of the movements for this change of roles, and in part repeat the instructions from the above four gestures.

Changing Positions

Using the energy of the waist and legs, along with the methods of sink the shoulders and hang the elbows, *B* then Withdraws and Entices to perform his Pushing. This then is Pushing with Advancing.

A, using the energy of the waist and legs, Neutralizes *B's* Push by bringing his left forearm slightly upwards and to the right to perform a Warding-Off circle. *A* having been the object of *B's* Pushing, begins Warding-Off and changes to Rolling-Back, with the left hand and arm performing the Rolling-Back. When Rolling-Back has been completed, *A* proceeds to perform Pressing.

A's left hand and arm make a half circular shape, just like embracing something, and the left hand attaches to the middle area between the right elbow and wrist. When perceiving the slightest movement of *B, A* uses the energy of the waist and legs, along with the method of sink the shoulders and hang the elbows, to perform a forward Pressing with Advancing towards *B's* chest cavity.

B then performs the Neutralizing right and left to *A,* and returns to Warding-Off. *A* will then be in the Pushing position.

A and *B* have now returned to their original starting positions.

Enclosed Stance

High Posturing

A   B

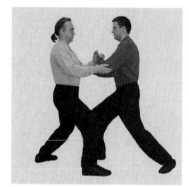
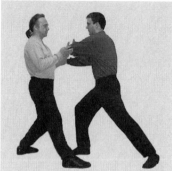
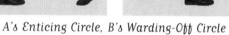

Starting Position   *A's Enticing Circle, B's Warding-Off Circle*

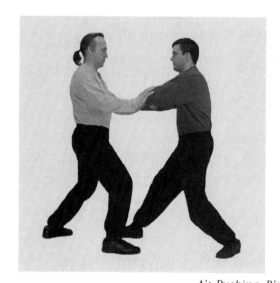
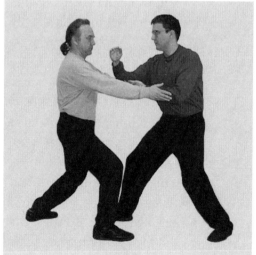

A's Pushing, B's Rolling-Back

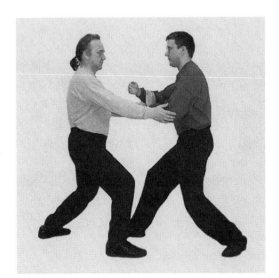 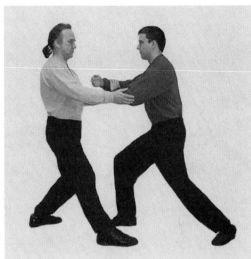

B's Pressing, A's Gazing-Right Neutralizing and Withdrawing Movement

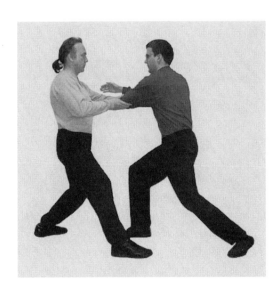 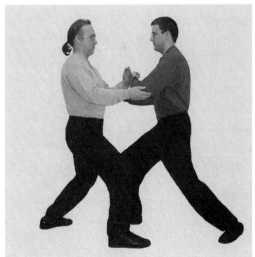

A's Looking-Left Neutralizing and Warding-Off
B's Circling to Stick and Adhere

The exercise continues with *B* now performing *A's* movements,
starting with the *Enticing Circle* and Advancing into *Push.*

Enclosed Stance

Medium Posturing

A   B

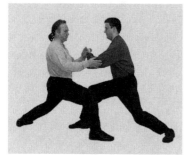 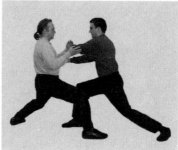

Starting Position   A's Enticing Circle, B's Warding-Off Circle

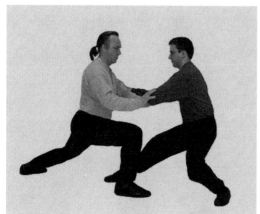 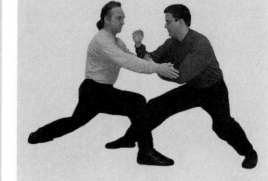

A's Pushing, B's Rolling-Back

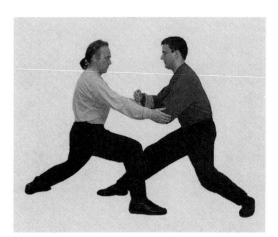
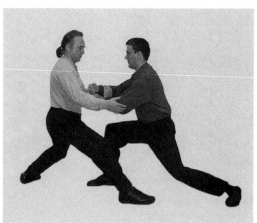

B's Pressing, A's Gazing-Right Neutralizing and Withdrawing Movement

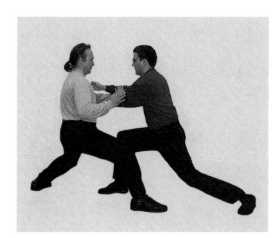
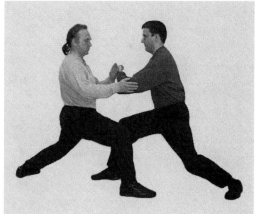

A's Looking-Left Neutralizing and Warding-Off
B's Circling to Stick and Adhere

The exercise continues with *B* now performing *A's* movements,
starting with the *Enticing Circle* and Advancing into *Push.*

Enclosed Stance

Low Posturing

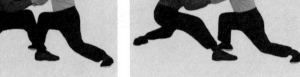

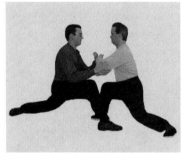
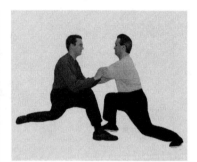

Starting Position   *A's Enticing Circle, B's Warding-Off Circle*

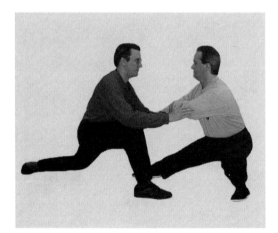
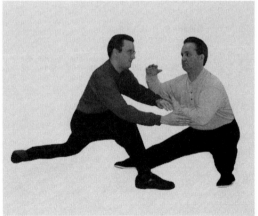

A's Pushing, B's Rolling-Back

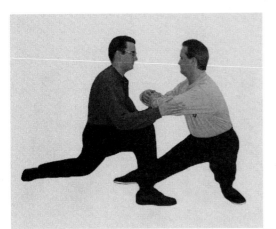 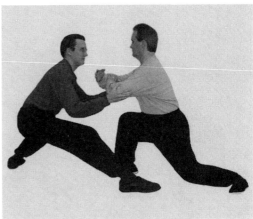

B's Pressing, A's Gazing-Right Neutralizing and Withdrawing Movement

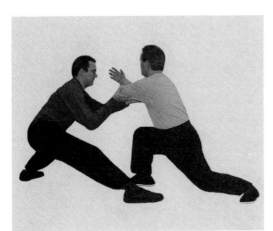 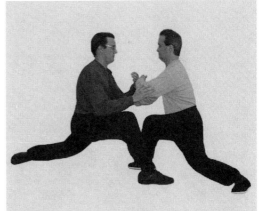

A's Looking-Left Neutralizing and Warding-Off
B's Circling to Stick and Adhere

The exercise continues with *B* now performing *A's* movements,
starting with the *Enticing Circle* and Advancing into *Push*.

Direct Stance

High Posturing

A   B

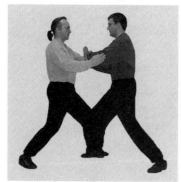
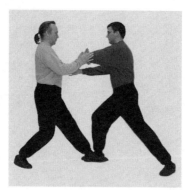

Starting Position   *A's Enticing Circle, B's Warding-Off Circle*

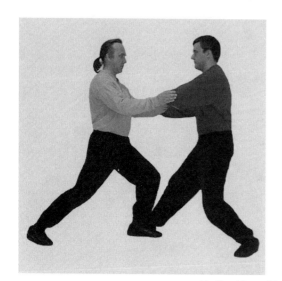
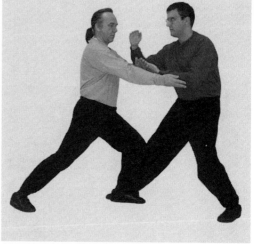

A's Pushing, B's Rolling-Back

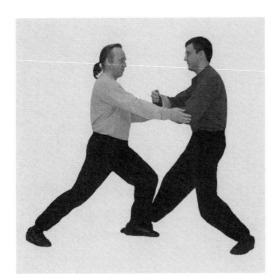
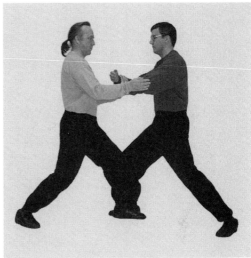

B's Pressing, A's Gazing-Right Neutralizing and Withdrawing Movement

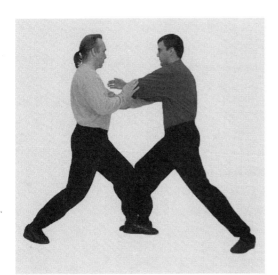
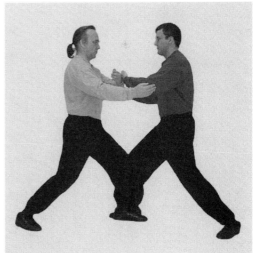

A's Looking-Left Neutralizing and Warding-Off
B's Circling to Stick and Adhere

The exercise continues with *B* now performing *A's* movements,
starting with the *Enticing Circle* and Advancing into *Push.*

Summary of the Four Skills
of Sensing-Hands in Fixed-Stance

Warding-Off, Rolling-Back, Pressing, and Pushing were previously distinguished as Advancing, Withdrawing, Looking-Left, Gazing-Right. There is also Fixed-Rooting.

What is Fixed-Rooting? In regards to application, Fixed-Rooting means that when there is Advancing, Withdrawing, Looking-Left, or Gazing-Right, Fixed-Rooting is contained within them. It is the Mind-Intent of your body's external center of balance which keeps you upright. Previous to *Issuing*, the *Internal Energy (Nei Chin)* must be produced in order to *Issue*, but first your posturing must have Fixed-Rooting. Then afterwards you can *Issue*. The appearance of this would, in analogy, be like the ringer inside a bell. When Neutralizing, the swaying movements to the left and right, are similar to ringing a bell. But when the Neutralizing arrives at *Issuing*, Fixed-Rooting is like that of the ringer. After acquiring Fixed-Rooting, you will be able to *Issue*. As a consequence, you will acquire the power of *Issuing Energy*, and not that of *Leaning* and *Discarding*. Therefore, Fixed-Rooting in regards to *Sensing-Hands* has a very important role.

As a reference:

> After performing Warding-Off, Rolling-Back is born.
> After Rolling-Back, Pressing is born.
> After Pressing, Neutralizing is born.
> After Neutralizing, Pushing is born.

Likewise,

> Pushing cannot be explained without the use of Warding-Off.
> Rolling-Back cannot be explained without the use of Pressing.
> Pressing cannot be explained without the use of Neutralizing.

Hence, Warding-Off, Rolling-Back, Pressing, and Pushing all reciprocally produce and destroy each other.

Translator's Comments
Neutralizing is to Warding-Off, Rolling-Back, Pressing, and Pushing as what Fixed-Rooting is to Advancing, Withdrawing, Looking-Left, and Gazing-Right—as Earth is to Metal, Fire, Water, and Wood.

Now, in regards to the time previous to Warding-Off, use of just the hand and arm is hardly adequate for producing even a little energy (*Chin*), so it will be without a good result. Without using the energy of the waist and legs, along with the Mind-Intent and *Ch'i*, it is not possible to apply Warding-Off correctly. So, previous to Warding-Off there must be incorporated a small circling of Neutralizing, if not, then it will be all too easy to produce an opposing energy.

In regards to the time previous to Rolling-Back, with the one hand facing towards the front, there must be Warding-Off. This will make the opponent's energy the object of *Inducing*, bringing the opponent forward. The hands then perform Rolling-Back to the opponent, making it possible to *Borrow* the opponent's energy. If not, then it will be all too easy to produce *Discarding* energy.

In regards to the time previous to Pressing, first make sure that the opponent has been the object of a completed Rolling-Back. After which, change to do Pressing. Your body should be brought near enough to the opponent to actually perform Shouldering (*Kao*). If not, then both parties will be too far apart, and you can be held at a distance, and so it will not be easy to acquire the opportunity to *Borrow* the opponent's energy, and it will be all too easy to have your center severed.

In regards to the time previous to Pushing, there must first be the Energy (*Chin*) of Neutralizing [Enticing Circle] to the rear. Neutralizing to the rear will cause the opponent's center of balance to incline towards the front. Then immediately take advantage of this opportunity by performing Advance. All this is to cause the opponent to fall on emptiness, which will in turn make it easier for you to *Borrow* his strength. If not, then certainly the opponent can seat his waist and secure his footing, causing his center of balance to be upright, and will be able to sink his *Ch'i* into the *Tan-T'ien*. How then can you perform Pushing?

Further, with either Pressing or Pushing, the body should not commit the defect of bending forward, as going too far forward will conversely make it all too easy for the opponent to *Borrow* your energy. In conjunction with this, the knees must not pass over the toes, and the elbows must not pass beyond the knees. For the body to remain intact, it must be held centered and upright, and this is accomplished by avoiding the corruptions of looking downwards *(bending)* and looking upwards *(leaning)*.

When performing *Sensing-Hands*, you must do away with externals in order to still the mind, concentrate the spirit, and to sink the *Ch'i* into the *Tan-T'ien*. To do so, proceed to incorporate the following principles:

> *Sink the shoulders and hang the elbows.*
> *Hollow the chest and raise the back.*
> *Retain a light and sensitive energy on top of the head.*
> *Keep the body centered and upright.*
> *Draw in the Wei-Lu.*
> *Relax the waist and pelvis.*
> *The waist, legs, and hands, along with the entire body,*
> *must act as one complete unit.*

These above conditions are particularly essential. Beyond these, in relation to the "line of direction" *(Fang Hsiang)*, the spirit of the eyes must gaze accordingly. This is likewise very important, just as Warding-Off must have an upwards gaze "line of direction." Rolling-Back must have a rearward gaze "line of direction." Pressing and Pushing must have a forward gaze "line of direction." On no account with the rearward "line of direction" of Rolling-Back would you look forward, nor with forward "line of direction" of Pressing would you look to the rear.

Translator's Comments

This *"line of direction"* means that the eyes follow the movement, which is created by the use of the energy of the waist and legs. Therefore, simply said, the eyes must follow the movements of the waist. The waist, accordingly, must follow the principle of *"the square-within-a-circle."* All of this is primarily concerned with disciplining the body to function as one unit.

Concerning the individual energies *(Chin)* of *Adhering, Sticking, Neutralizing, Seizing,* and *Issuing,* you should read and carefully examine the section titled *Discourses on the Intrinsic Energies,* and the sections on the breathing procedures should also be read over carefully.* So that I will not have to keep making repeated references to these interior materials, I will render a brief summary below.

Relative to learning the *Four Skills of Sensing-Hands in Fixed-Stance,* the techniques of Warding-Off, Rolling-Back, Pressing, and Pushing are central and you should undertake very serious study of them. The waist and legs especially must be trained so that each of the abilities of *Adhering, Sticking, Joining,* and *Following* can make the body natural, compliant, open, expanded, without hindrance, and devoid of even a fraction of External Muscular Force *(Li).* Once this is achieved, as soon as you are affected by something, you respond immediately. Gesture by gesture, each becoming completely rounded out and with no projections produced.

To speak on this further, suppose that a student was able to train the *Four Skills* until each gesture was completely rounded out. Within this no projections are produced, with no severance and no entanglements also. More so, the entire body must be relaxed and opened, so that later the waist and legs function as one unit. Then when performing *Sensing-Hands,* and the hands begin to interact with the opponent, you are immediately compelled to come out. When this happens you should produce a response similar to something being repelled out from a spinning wheel. This means that when you meet with an opponent you should be circular, rather than both parties just running into each other and so creating resistance. If so, you will be unable to bring about a counteraction.

Hence, the gesture-by-gesture movements of T'ai Chi Ch'uan should

---

* Discourses on the Intrinsic Energies has been translated by me. See *The Intrinsic Energies of T'ai Chi Ch'uan.* In regards to breathing, see *Cultivating the Ch'i.*

likewise each embody a circular appearance. Taking the example from this, it is an exceptional student who when performing the *Four Skills* can to the utmost be circular and rounded out, and so be able to use the whole body as one unit. Consequently, there will then be no occasion in which you will adopt to the opponent's slight-of-hand techniques, as it will be your feet and legs that will respond to the opponent.

Translator's Comments
The *T'ai Chi Ch'uan Treatise* states, *"When the body is in a state of disorder and confusion, correct this by adjusting the waist and legs."* Meaning, never try to wrestle or force your way out of a bad situation with the hands; rather, rely on the movements and adjustments of the waist and legs.

The above should be regarded as the stationary training methods of the *Four Skills of Sensing-Hands in Fixed-Stance* methods of Warding-Off, Rolling-Back, Pressing, and Pushing. However, when your skills are deepened, it will be unnecessary to make use of these stationary procedures. For in *Warding-Off, Rolling-Back, Pressing, Pushing, Pulling, Splitting, Elbowing, Shouldering, Opening, Closing, Enticing, Neutralizing, Seizing,* and *Issuing*—what posturing, what gesturing, are not contained within them?

When you are being attacked, *follow*. When you are being Neutralized, *follow*. If attacked high, *gaze high*. If attacked low, *respond low*. If attacked by Advance, *seize the opportunity with Advance*. If attacked with Withdraw, *follow-step with Withdraw*. Always follow when the situation is tightly closed off, but seeing a crack immediately Advance, for it will be far worse if your energy *(Chin)* is severed.

The techniques and principles of *San-shou and Ta-Lu* could also be interjected here, to either defense or offense, which enable you to learn how to completely adapt to the changes and accord with all circumstances, so when seeing the conditions, you move in perfect response to them. By all means seek to clearly distinguish the Substantial and Insubstantial—the *Yin* and *Yang*. Cause yourself to be able to follow those conditions, and so put the opponent far into the background, yet never parting from the four words of *Adhering, Sticking, Joining,* and *Following*.

The Four Skills of Sensing-Hands in Active-Steps

Warding-Off, Rolling-Back, Pressing, and Pushing

In relation to *Fixed-Stance Sensing-Hands*, train so that the waist and legs acquire the abilities of *Adhering, Sticking, Joining,* and *Following.* From this the body methods and stepping methods are capable of adapting and according with the opponent's spontaneously, capable of responding to the changes and following all circumstances, so that afterwards there is not even a trace remaining of External Muscular Force *(Li).* Then proceed to the next stage and begin training *Active-Step Sensing-Hands,* which will create the conditions for the entire body, both the upper and lower, to function as one unit.

How to begin the actual stepping for *Neutralizing* and *Issuing* to each person? The training procedure for both persons is to initially engage in just the turning and circling gestures with *Fixed-Stance* gesturing, then begin applying the hands and feet with *Active-Step* methods for Advancing, Withdrawing, Looking-Left, Gazing-Right, and Fixed-Rooting, whereby each person can train to Close Off *(Ho)* a strike. Whether this is done fast or slow, the movements must be kept level and even. Under no circumstance can the hands be fast and the feet slow, or the hands slow and the feet fast. Likewise, if the feet have not yet arrived, then the hands must not arrive beforehand, or if the hands have not yet arrived, then the feet could not already be there either.

Methods of the Four Skills
in Active-Steps

Instructions for Right-Style Training
Active-Steps
High Posturing, and Enclosed Stance

Starting Position
The stance methods here are the same as with *Fixed-Stance Sensing-Hands*, and can be performed using either *Enclosed* or *Direct Stances*.

Both parties stand opposite of one another, each bringing their right foot forward.

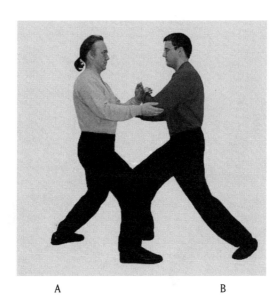

A   B

Translator's Comments
The particulars of the movements here are identical to those of the *Four Skills of Fixed-Stance Sensing-Hands* given previously, so they need not be repeated here. The only difference is, obviously, the stepping movements.

The instructions here are shown according to the gestures of Enclosed Stance, the Direct Stance is shown photo-
graphically only.

A's Enticing Circle with Advance-Step,
and B's Warding-Off Circle with Withdraw-Step

When Withdrawing into the rear leg and Enticing, A picks up his right
foot, Advances it one half step to the front, and Slide-Steps his left foot
one half step as well. At the same time, B performs the Warding-Off
Circle, picks up his left foot, and when A steps forward, B Withdraws to
the rear one half step, and Slide-Steps back with his right foot.

B, after having been the object of Enticing and stepping back to
Neutralize, then seats the waist, relaxes the pelvis, seats the legs, and
Neutralizes towards the rear.

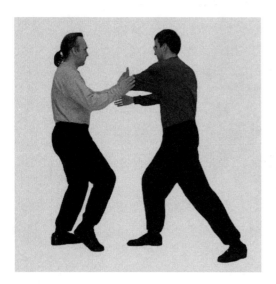 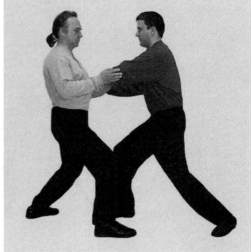

A's Pushing with Advance-Step, and B's Warding-Off and Rolling-Back with Withdraw-Step

After A's Enticing Pushing has been Neutralized, A picks up the left foot and steps one step forward—this can be viewed from either an offense or defense perspective—to perform Pushing with Advance-Step. B, maintaining his Warding-Off position of the hands and arms, Withdraw-Steps back one step with the right foot.

A then continues his Pushing by picking up his right foot and Advance-Stepping one more step forward. B then Withdraw-Steps one step back with his left foot, then seats the waist, relaxes the pelvis, seats the legs, and Neutralizes towards the left corner by Rolling-Back.

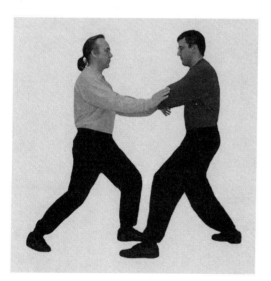 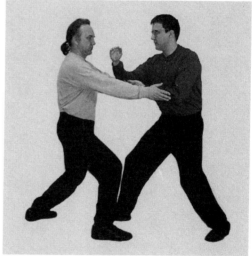

Translator's Comments

Although Chen Kung says this exercise can be practiced with one-step, two-step, three-step, or more movements, the instructions refer to taking two steps so that the Rolling-Back, Pressing, and Neutralizing movements end up in the same arm and leg positions as in the Fixed-Stance exercise.

In the above gesture, if A's Push takes place in only one Advance-Step, B's Rolling-Back would still occur to the left, but his left leg would be forward instead of his right.

As you become proficient in this exercise, you should practice these movements with varying steps to see the different possibilities and train your waist and legs to handle them without your having to think about it.

B's Pressing with Advance-Step, and A's Gazing-Right Neutralizing with Withdraw-Step

After Withdraw-Stepping to perform Rolling-Back, B changes into Pressing by picking up the left foot and Advance-Stepping one step forward. A, likewise, Withdraw-Steps back with the right foot while performing Gazing-Right Neutralizing.

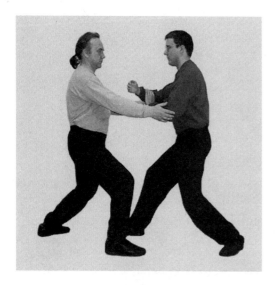 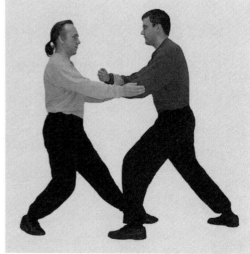

B's Circling to Stick and Adhere with Advance-Step, and A's Looking-Left Neutralizing and Warding-Off with Withdraw-Step

B, following A's movements, Advance-Steps with his right foot and circles his waist and hands to the right, ending up in the starting position, Sticking with his left hand to A's left hand, which has moved into a Warding-Off position, and Adhering with his right hand to A's elbow.

Having Neutralized *B's* Pressing and Advance-Step, *A* Withdraw-Steps one step back with the left foot while performing Looking-Left Neutralizing and bringing his left arm downward, before raising the arm upward into Warding-Off and Advancing into the forward leg. He is then back in the starting position as well.

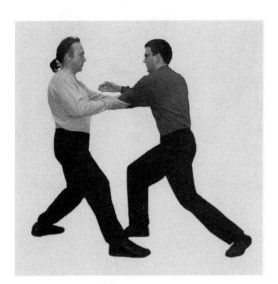 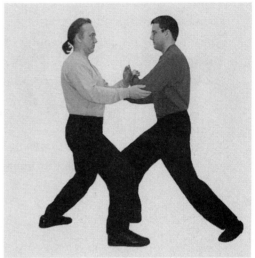

Translator's Comments

The positions now change so that *B* will be performing the Pushing and Neutralizing movements, and *A* performing the Rolling-Back and Pressing ones.

The gestures follow a pattern wherein the person who is Pushing Advances two-and-a-half steps forward, and then Neutralizes two steps back to the original starting point. Then, as the roles reverse and he is now Warding-Off and Rolling-Back, he takes two-and-a-half steps backward, before stepping two steps forward again by Pressing and moving back into Push, his original starting position.

This is the *Right-Style* for *Active-Steps*. The *Left-Style* is performed in the same manner except the legs and arm positions are opposite.

Enclosed Stance

A   B

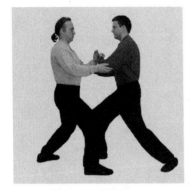 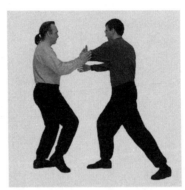 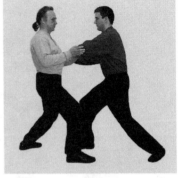

Starting Position

A's Enticing Circle with Advance-Step (1/2 step forward, South),
B's Warding-Off Circle with Withdraw-Step (1/2 step backward)

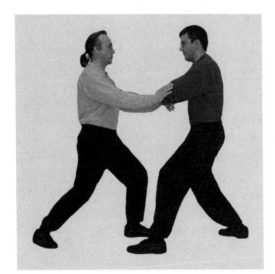 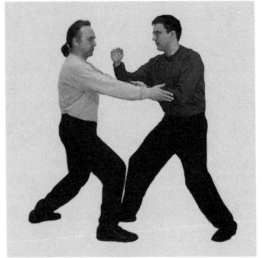

A's Pushing with Advance-Step (2 steps forward, South),
B's Warding-Off and Rolling-Back with Withdraw-Step (2 steps backward)

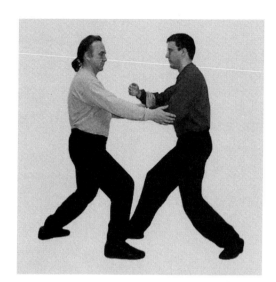 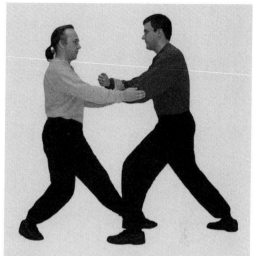

Switch Directions
B's Pressing with Advance-Step (1 step forward, North)
A's Gazing-Right Neutralizing with Withdraw-Step (1 step backward)

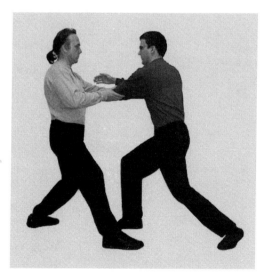 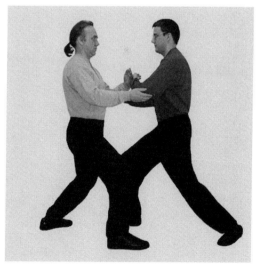

B's Circling to Stick and Adhere with Advance-Step (1 step forward, North)
A's Looking-Left Neutralizing and Warding-Off with Withdraw-Step (1 step backward)

The exercise continues with *B* now performing *A's* movements, starting with the *Enticing Circle with Advance-Step* and going into *Pushing with Advance-Step*.

Instructions for Active-Steps
in the Direct Stance

When practicing Active-Stepping in Direct Stance, the person who is Advancing steps to the inside of the opponent's leg, while the opponent, who is Withdrawing, *Adheres* his leg to the outside of the incoming opponent's leg.

When Advancing, you step to the inside of an opponent's leg to create an opportunity for affecting the opponent's knee and leg, making it easy to upset his center of balance. Stepping to the inside will also prevent the opponent from either kicking you or kneeing you in the groin.

When Withdrawing, you *Adhere* your leg to the outside of the incoming opponent's leg so that you can either sweep his foot or affect the outside of his knee to destroy his center of balance.

Direct Stance

A   B

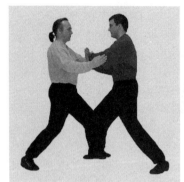
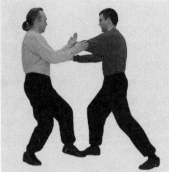

Starting Position

A's Enticing Circle with Advance-Step (1/2 step forward, South),
B's Warding-Off Circle with Withdraw-Step (1/2 step backward)

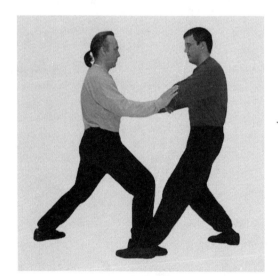
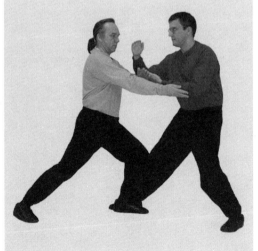

A's Pushing with Advance-Step (2 steps forward, South),
B's Warding-Off and Rolling-Back with Withdraw-Step (2 steps backward)

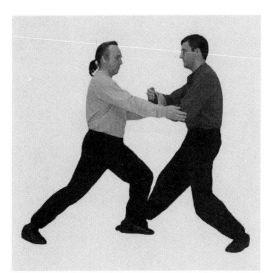 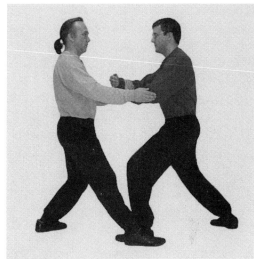

Switch Directions
B's Pressing with Advance-Step (1 step forward, North)
A's Gazing-Right Neutralizing with Withdraw-Step (1 step backward)

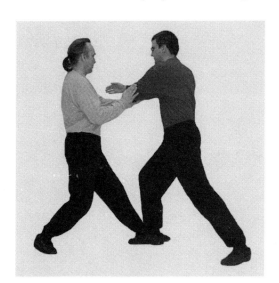 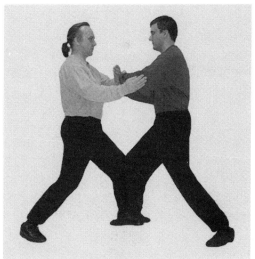

B's Circling to Stick and Adhere with Advance-Step (1 step forward, North)
A's Looking-Left Neutralizing and Warding-Off with Withdraw-Step (1 step backward)

The exercise continues with *B* now performing *A's* movements, starting with the *Enticing Circle with Advance-Step* and going into *Pushing with Advance-Step*.

Summary of the Four Skills
of Sensing-Hands in Active-Steps

Advancing means that two-and-a-half steps are taken. Withdrawing means that two-and-a-half steps are also taken, with both persons performing Warding-Off, Rolling-Back, Pressing, Pushing, and Neutralizing. Each movement is just like that within *Fixed-Stance Sensing-Hands*, yet they must, gesture by gesture, be clearly distinguished, with the posturing being followed and adapted to the applications. These stepping procedures are the initial training, but for those whose skills deepen need not maintain these prescribed number of steps.

In relation to the older Yang Family-style of *Active-Step Sensing-Hands*, and that of the above description are not quite the same. To step forward for Advancing means first stepping back in conjunction with the going forward; to step back for Withdrawing means first stepping to the front before Withdrawing back.

Translator's Comments
This means that before stepping forward (Advancing) there would be a half step to the back first with the opposite foot. With each step to the rear (Withdrawing) there would first be a half step to the front. These instructions forego the above older version of stepping.

Advancing and Withdrawing can be either two steps, four steps, or even six steps. Any of these will suffice. Yet, you must take the waist and legs to be the pivotal axis of all the movements. The substantial and insubstantial must be clearly discriminated when the stepping is mobilized. In the event of the two persons performing the *Direct Stances*, the first step is Advancing. The foot that is Withdrawing should then be positioned on the outer side of the Advancing opponent's foot.

Translator's Comments
The Pushing and Pressing movements can either be performed with one step for each, or two steps for Pushing and then two more for Pressing, as well as taking three steps for

Pushing and three more for Pressing. The opposite person will also make the same number steps when Withdrawing as the person Advancing. The half step at the beginning however remains the same no matter how many steps are used later for Pushing and Pressing.

All the movements described above are more difficult to perform than *Fixed-Stance Sensing-Hands*. Along with *Active-Step Sensing-Hands* are the regulative procedures of keeping the body centered and upright; retaining a light and sensitive energy on top of the head; hollowing the chest and raising the back; sinking the shoulders and hanging the elbows; sinking the *Ch'i* into the *Tan-T'ien*; drawing in the *Wei-Lu*; relaxing the waist and pelvis; and beyond these, the entire body must function as one unit.

Afterwards you should arrive at a certain level, such as the inhaling and exhaling of the internal *Ch'i*, along with the correct manner of fixing the attention on the breath. However, during your initial training just seek to keep the breath as natural as possible. There is also no need to give any consideration to the external styles of breathing, as they will not bring about any proficiency of inhaling and exhaling of the internal *Ch'i*.

Aside from externally training the waist, legs, hands, and feet, the upper and lower parts of the body must act as one unit. It will then be possible for the *Ch'i* to function in a prolonged manner. This will enable the body to endure the hard work of training and repair any acquired insufficiencies needed for training *Fixed-Stance Sensing-Hands*.

Active-Step Sensing-Hands is also divided into three types of posturing (*Chia Tzu*)—High, Middle, and Low. The beginning stage is to train the High Posturing (*Kao Chia Tzu*); intermediates train the Middle Posturing (*Chung Chia Tzu*), and then afterwards the Low Posturing (*Ti Chia Tzu*) can be trained. After becoming accustomed to the sequences and order of the exercises, you may then simultaneously practice these Three Posturings.

Translator's Comments

High Posturing is a normal stance with the knees slightly bent. The distance between the feet is shoulder-width, and the length is two foot lengths to the front.

Middle Posturing is a lower seated position. The distance between the feet is still shoulder-width, but the length is three foot lengths to the front.

Lower Posturing is a very low squatting position. The distance between the two feet is one foot length wider than shoulder-width, and the length is five foot lengths to the front. See pages 148–49 for illustrations showing the Three Posturings.

In regards as to the occasion when performing *Active-Step Sensing-Hands*, and aside from the aspects of Advancing, Withdrawing, Looking-Left, and Gazing-Right, the Mind-Intent *(Yi)* and *Ch'i* must unite and the eyes must gaze intently outwards. In relation to Fixed-Rooting, you must give added attention to it. If not, the *Neutralizing* or *Issuing* of an opponent would be impossible, and it will be very easy for your center of balance to become inclined to one side.

Therefore, within an old T'ai Chi Ch'uan document it says:

"When Withdrawing, circling is easy, but Advancing and circling is much more difficult. The waist and legs must not separate either before or after (the circling), for it would then be difficult to maintain your center by staying attached to the ground to hold your stance. Withdrawing is easy, Advancing is difficult—carefully investigate this thoroughly."

This above verse is referring to the practice of the moving exercises *(Active-Steps)*, not for the standing ones *(Fixed-Stance)*. To the body, Advancing and Withdrawing are side-by-side equals. The ability to be like this is as though pressing on a water mill, either fast or slow. The clouds, dragons, wind, and fire all revolve and move about equally. You should also seek to make use of these Heavenly Vessels *(T'ien Pan)*, so that in the course of time it will all naturally just come out.

Translator's Comments
T'ien Pan could also be translated as "Nature's Vessels." The idea being that T'ai Chi draws its principles and techniques from the natural movements and functions of nature. Here, the analogies mean to move as soft and carefree as a cloud, as binding and invisible as a dragon, as supple and strong as the wind, and as penetrating and destructive as fire.

You can hopefully see from all the above how important the *Active-Step Sensing-Hands* truly is. In relation to the minute particulars of the movements themselves, it is impossible to acquire them all without a secret oral transmission of the teachings.

Translator's Comments
Although the instructions and words of this book can greatly enhance your Sensing-Hands skills, at some point you will need to seek a qualified teacher who can not only verbalize, but also demonstrate these teachings to you so that you can fully grasp and assimilate them. The bulk of the material contained here has to be empirically understood, not just read.

Those who just practice these exercises for ordinary martial art use are unaware of the correctness and truth of these original writings, and that it should be advocated as a unique and clever means for strengthening the nation. Do not reject the careful attention given to the details in these writings, for contained within them are all the necessary instructions to accomplish this end.

Translator's Comments
The statements, ideas, and concepts presented within this book are as profound and insightful as those made in *Sun Tzu's Art of War* or the *Book of Changes* itself. There is no question that this work could be used, with the right interpretations, to strengthen not only a person's character, but the better governing of a nation as well.

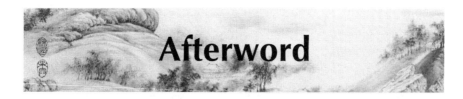

Afterword

This book has primarily provided detailed instructions for the ten main Right-Style stances of *T'ui-Shou*—the preliminary Eight Styles of Sensing-Hands exercises, and the Fixed-Stance and Active-Steps exercises of the Four Skills of Sensing-Hands (Warding-Off, Rolling-Back, Pressing, and Pushing). Even though the instructions given here are only for the Right-Style stances, the Left-Style stances must also be trained. All the exercises in this book should eventually be practiced in the following eight variations:

1) Fixed-Stance *(Ting Pu)* with Enclosed Stances *(Ho Pu)*

2) Fixed-Stance *(Ting Pu)* with Direct Stances *(Shun Pu)*

3) Active-Steps (*Huo Pu*) with Enclosed Stances *(Ho Pu)*

4) Active-Steps *(Hou Pu)* with Direct Stances *(Shun Pu)*

5) All Fixed-Stances and Active-Steps with *Cheng* movements (horizontal-level gesturing).

6) All of the above are to be practiced in the Three Posturings— High, Medium, and Low positions.

7) All of the above Fixed-Stance and Active-Steps with *Tao* movements (vertical wave-like gesturing moving from Low to High). Since *Tao* vertical movements work from Low to High positions, the Three Posturings are inherently incorporated into them.

8) Free-Style movements, drawn from any of the above methods.

Beginners would be well advised to practice the above methods in the following order and not proceed to the next method until having gained some proficiency.

- First train all the exercises in Fixed-Stance with Enclosed Stances and *Cheng* movements in High and then Medium posturings, learning both the Right and Left Styles.
- Afterwards, proceed to train all the exercises of Active-Steps with Enclosed Stances and *Cheng* movements in High and then Medium posturings, learning both the Right and Left Styles.
- Once these are accomplished, begin practicing all the exercises of Fixed-Stance with Direct Stances and *Cheng* movements in High and Medium posturings, learning both the Right and Left Styles.
- Next train all the exercises of Active-Steps with Direct Stances and *Cheng* movements in High and then Medium posturings, learning both the Right and Left Styles.
- Then train all the exercises, Enclosed and Direct Stances, with both Fixed-Stance and Active-Steps, and *Cheng* movements with just Low posturing, in both the Right and Left Styles.
- After training all these variations, apply the *Tao* movements to all the above exercises.
- Train all the exercises in the Three Positionings, the relationship of *A* and *B*'s front feet to each other, for both Enclosed and Direct Stances.

Enclosed Stance

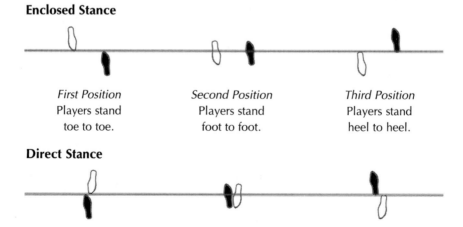

First Position
Players stand
toe to toe.

Second Position
Players stand
foot to foot.

Third Position
Players stand
heel to heel.

Direct Stance

Train all the exercises in the First Position and then the Second, but do not attempt the Third until both partners are proficient in the first two, otherwise too much tension may be applied.

Enclosed Bow Stances in the Three Posturings and Three Positionings

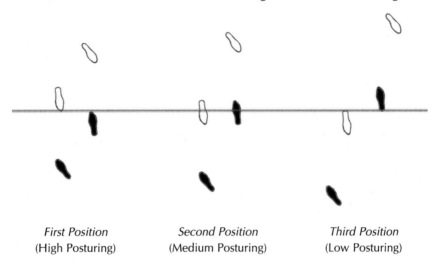

First Position	*Second Position*	*Third Position*
(High Posturing)	(Medium Posturing)	(Low Posturing)

Direct Bow Stances

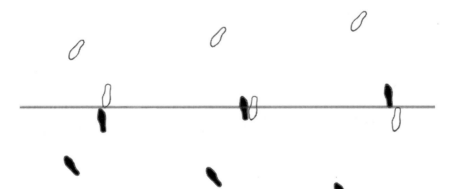

- Lastly, train Free-Style Sensing-Hands, which involves using any of the exercises and their variations in an open, unstructured manner, moving from one into another in no set pattern but just responding to each other's movements.

Though it is simply stated in a few paragraphs, the above training is an enormous—yet rewarding—undertaking. It requires years of practice to accomplish a high level of proficiency in all the variations of Sensing-Hands. Nevertheless, just take your time, proceed step-by-step, and gradually you will experience improvements and breakthroughs.

Golfers, for example, don't think about the years of practice they put into improving their game, they mostly deal with what is happening to them in the present. They look forward to getting out there and playing. If you take the attitude of a golfer, or of anyone who is strongly committed to a practice, art, or hobby, and apply that to your Sensing-Hands training, you can't fail to improve—and to stick with it.

If the art of T'ai Chi was simple to perform and easy to acquire it would not be worth anyone's effort because it would be limited in skills, benefits, attainments, wisdom, and experience. T'ai Chi means "the supreme ultimate," or "the highest of ultimates," and whatever that *ultimate* is, it is surely beyond comprehension and beyond the scope of this or any other writing.

Suggested Reading

Although there are many valuable works on T'ai Chi not mentioned here, the following suggested readings relate well to the information presented in this book. I am not certain, however, if all of them are still in print, but for serious adherents the following works will help them greatly in their practice.

Advanced Yang Style
Tai Chi Chuan
Volume One, Tai Chi Theory
and Tai Chi Jing
By Dr. Yang Jwing-Ming
YMAA, 1986

Advanced Yang Style
Tai Chi Chuan
Volume Two, Martial Applications
By Dr. Yang Jwing-Ming
YMAA, 1986

Chen Style Taijiquan
By Feng Zhiqiang and Feng Dabiao
Hai Feng Publishing Co., 1984

Cheng Tzu's Thirteen Treatises
on T'ai Chi Ch'uan
By Cheng Man-ch'ing
Translated by Benjamin Pang Jeng
Lo and Martin Inn
North Atlantic Books, 1985

Chinese Boxing
Masters and Methods
By Robert W. Smith
North Atlantic Books, 1990

Cultivating the Ch'i:
The Secrets of Energy and Vitality
Compiled and Translated
by Stuart Alve Olson
Dragon Door Publications, 1993

The Intrinsic Energies
of T'ai Chi Ch'uan
Translated by Stuart Alve Olson
Dragon Door Publications, 1994

Lee's Modified Tai Chi for Health
By Lee Ying-arng
Melissa Enterprises, 1968

Lost T'ai-chi Classics
from the Late Ching Dynasty
By Douglas Wile
State University of New York
(SUNY) Press, 1996

Practical Use of Tai Chi Chuan:
Its Applications & Variations
By Yeung (Yang) Sau Chung
Tai Chi Co., 1976

Tai Chi Ch'uan:
The Technique of Power
By Tem Horwitz and Susan
Kimmelman with H.H. Liu
Chicago Review Press, 1976

T'ai Chi Ch'uan for Health
and Self-Defense:
Philosophy and Practice
By Master T.T. Liang
Vintage Books, 1977

The Tao of T'ai Chi Ch'uan:
Way to Rejuvenation
By Jou, Tsung Hwa
T'ai Chi Foundation, 1980

T'ai Chi Ch'uan Principles
and Practice
By C.K. Chu
Sunflower Press, 1981

T'ai Chi for Two
By Paul Crompton
Shambala, 1996

Tui Shou & San Shou
in T'ai Chi Ch'uan
By Yiu Kwong
Self-Published, 1980

Wu Style Tai Chi Chuan Tui Shou
By Ma Yueh Liang and Zee Wen
Shanghai Book Co., Ltd., 1986

Wu Style Taijiquan
By Wang Pei-sheng and Zeng Weiqi
Hai Feng Publishing Co., 1983

Yang Style Taijiquan
Edited by Yu Shengquan
Hai Feng Publishing Co., 1988

About the Translator

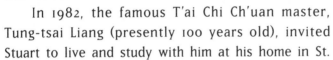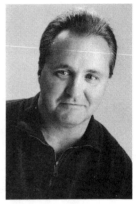

In 1979, as a resident of *Ju Lai Sôu* monastery at the City of Ten-Thousand Buddhas in Talmage, California, Stuart began learning the Chinese language and studying Buddhist philosophy, taking formal refuge in Buddhism from Ch'an Master Hsuan Hua.

In 1982, the famous T'ai Chi Ch'uan master, Tung-tsai Liang (presently 100 years old), invited Stuart to live and study with him at his home in St. Cloud, Minnesota. Stuart was the only student ever granted this honor. While staying in Master Liang's home for over six years, Stuart studied both T'ai Chi Ch'uan and Chinese language under Master Liang's tutelage. Since then Stuart has traveled extensively throughout the United States with Master Liang assisting him in teaching. Stuart has also taught in Canada, Hong Kong, and Indonesia, and has traveled throughout Asia. He has also studied massage in both Taiwan and Indonesia.

Stuart presently lives in the Twin Cities, Minnesota. He teaches *Yi T'ai Chi* (a 64-Posture Yang Style T'ai Chi Form based entirely on the images of the *Book of Changes—Yi-Ching*), related Yang Style forms and weapons, *Eight Brocades Seated Qi-Gong,* and *Chin Ku Sung* massage.

Stuart continues to travel and teach, as well as translate and compile Asian related books. If you wish to contact him, or receive a detailed workshop list and seminar update, please send a letter to the following address:

P.O. Box 18294
Minneapolis, MN 55418